15 STEPS TO HEALTHY LIVING

15 STEPS TO HEALTHY LIVING

DR. GORDON FIMREITE

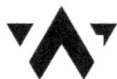

WASHINGTON SUITE
PUBLISHING

Chicago, IL

Washington Suite Publishing, Chicago, IL.
Printed in the United States of America – November, 2017

This publication contains the opinions and ideas of its author. It is intended to provide helpful and informative material on the subjects addressed in the publication. The reader should consult his or her medical professional before adopting any of the suggestions in this book or drawing inferences from it. The author and publisher specifically disclaim all responsibility for any liability, loss, or risk, personal or otherwise, that is incurred as a consequence, directly or indirectly of the use or application of any of the contents of this book. This book is not intended as a substitute for the medical advice of physicians.

Book cover by D. Grbic
Photos by Zoe McKenzie Photography
Exercise Diagrams by Manoj Bhargav, M. Rao and CL Suen

www.drfimreite.com/15StepsToHealthyLiving

_____

ISBN-13: 978-0-9995480-0-4 (Paperback)
ISBN-13: 978-0-9995480-1-1 (E-book)
Library of Congress Control Number: 2017916226

This book is dedicated to my parents,
my grandparents and for all those who have
paved the way for healthy living.

Contents

Preface

I'm fascinated with healthy living and longevity. Not only because of my own interest and professional studies in health and wellness, but also because of my grandmother who lived a healthy life into her 100's.

Until age 95, she lived in her own apartment. At this time, she felt she wanted to live among other people her own age and moved to an assisted living nursing home. But within a few weeks and in her own light-hearted way found it "too depressing" being around all those "old people" and she moved back into her own apartment.

At age 102, she was still living in her own apartment, preparing her own healthy meals, washing her dishes and doing most things you and I would do. Possessing a great sense of humor and zest for life, she continued to laugh and enjoy life until she passed away at 105.

In her later years in life, I sat down with her and asked her how she approached life -- her basic attitude, her diet and what she thought accounted for her longevity. If there's a secret to living such a long and healthy life, I wanted to hear it from someone in their 100's.

She told me that while heredity was a factor "... just as important is my diet. I eat healthy foods. And I keep my mind and body active."

In that one sentence, she summarized the life habits that lead to a long healthy life. That was the secret I was looking for, though I didn't realize it until after I started writing this book.

And while she didn't say it specifically, I knew that her attitude was also a factor. She didn't see herself in her 100's. Her dreams were of being able to run and play in the fields as she did as a child growing up on a farm.

If everyone applied these simple living habits of eating healthy and keeping the mind and body active, longevity would run in everyone's family.

Introduction

Eating from the Earth

My sprightly grandmother was raised and spent most of her life on a farm in Wisconsin. Inevitably, she consumed natural foods that included raw, unpasteurized milk, butter and cream. And though this meant that she consumed much animal fat, research shows that fats are actually vital for good health if they come from pastured cows.

She was however lactose intolerant, meaning she had difficulty with digesting lactose (milk sugar) and therefore restricted her intake of cheese and dairy products.

What dairy she did consume was unpasteurized, which is healthier than pasteurized milk and easier for those who are lactose intolerant to digest. Pasteurization heats milk at high temperatures to kill unwanted bacteria and, in the process kills beneficial bacteria called probiotics which we'll talk about in detail later in the book. Pasteurization also damages the enzymes needed for digestion along with vitamins and minerals.

She also regularly ate garden raised fruits and vegetables, such as carrots, cucumbers, peppers, parsley, tomatoes, different kinds of lettuce, apples, pears and blueberries, along with canned goods.

Rotation Method

The food my grandmother ate was grown with the traditional rotation method, which is what farmers did when she was a child and which keeps the soil's minerals from depleting. For example, if you raised tomatoes in a certain area of the garden, the next year you would raise a different produce like broccoli. The farmer would continue this rotation cycle for six years.

After six years of rotating after each year's yields, they would plant nothing on that section of the garden for the seventh year. They would give it a year to rest, much like the 7th day (Sunday) is historically a day of rest. They would do the same with the yields from which they fed the farm animals. They would rotate the corn to wheat fields from year to year and after rotating it for six years, they would give that land a rest. They found the land would yield higher quality produce as well as preserve the top soil.

At the age of 102, I asked her about her diet. My grandmother's food selection wasn't based on longevity, but rather the knowledge she knew at that time as being healthy. We will give suggestions on food selections for optimal health later. Since my grandmother was raised on a farm in a rural community, she grew up eating foods produced from the farm until later in her life. She was raised during a time when processed and fast foods were not an integral part of society. This is a partial list of what she ate regularly in her later life when processed and fast foods were readily available.

Breakfast: Lactate milk, 2 eggs with ½ yolk and oatmeal. She tried not to exceed 3 egg yolks per week.

Lunch, Snacks: Warm lactate milk; potatoes; 12 grain bread; fruit jam (all natural) - black cherry, black berry and strawberry; ground horseradish root for flavoring; wheat germ with whole wheat; shredded wheat; Cheerios cereal added to boiling water along with lactate milk; glass of ruby red grapefruit frozen juice; puffed rice; bananas, apples, pears, peaches, plums, cherries, oranges, mandarin oranges.

Dinner: Chicken soup; oatmeal with a potato and rice; chicken; ½ teaspoon tuna fish (sparingly because of the salt); broccoli, celery, carrots, cauliflower, lettuce, rutabagas.

Grinding Her Food

In addition to what she ate, my grandmother ground her food because she only had 12 teeth. This was actually a blessing as food already ground is easier for the body to digest. Plants are covered with cellulose, a protective cell wall. To release the enzyme cellulose in the plant, we must first break down the cellulose. To do this we need to chew our food to a creamy consistency. Few do. Most people chew once or twice per mouthful. Even if you did chew vigorously, you could not chew each seed in a strawberry long enough to break it down. Breaking down the food ahead of time solves this problem so you get more nutrients from your food. This is one of the reasons why juicing and blending of raw food is so healthy for us and has become so popular.

Use It or Lose It

In addition to healthy eating, my grandmother's wisdom included keeping her sharp brain active. Her advice was to "keep busy, keep busy, keep busy... Keep your brain busy... You have to think... just like exercising to get big muscles, you have to use your mind to get more brain power." Keeping your brain "busy, busy, busy..." fosters what we would now call neuroplasticity, the ability of the brain, even in old age, to keep growing and rewiring as long as you use it.

And use it my grandmother did. She enjoyed crossword puzzles and she loved reading. She always had reading material at hand as reading was "relaxing" she would read a little, think a little and then read more. If she had a strenuous day, she would read before settling in for the evening. She especially enjoyed true stories. Reading the Bible regularly gave her purpose for living.

Get Outside & Soak Up the Sun

My grandmother stayed physically active. She enjoyed especially going outdoors for walks in the sunshine. Even before longevity studies confirmed the importance of vitamin D for health and longevity she recognized that exposing her arms and face to the sun gave her natural vitamin D.

People Who Love People

Social interaction is an important part of longevity and healthy living and my grandmother, with her love of people and enjoyment of giving to others, fully took advantage of social engagement. She would give away one of her favorite books to the new people she would meet. Every time she went to church, she would sit in a different area by someone new and give them a book. It was her way to introduce herself. She loved telling stories and meeting new people. She also stressed the importance of keeping in touch with people.

Added Up

It's fascinating how much the way she lived her life parallels what research studies are showing to contribute to healthy living and longevity. She ate nutritious foods, exercised, spent time in the sun to get her needed vitamin D, relaxed to handle stress, socialized, enjoyed humor, and had a purpose for living through her faith in God.

Unfortunately, not everyone has my grandmother's wisdom. Many people today eat poorly, exercise rarely, spend more time passively in front of a screen than actively doing mind games, socialize more on Facebook than out in the community, and lack purpose in their lives. Nor does everyone feel motivated to turn their lives around to a healthy lifestyle. This really hit home when I began giving speeches. People would share how difficult, even overwhelming it was to begin healthy habits and stick with them. During one of my speeches, someone yelled, "You have to die of something!" The audience burst into laughter.

I thought I was passionately sharing ways to change daily habits and optimize health and add to a longer, more vibrant life. In truth I was overwhelming the audience with healthy tips and health concepts. Little wonder all they could think of was, "I can't give up my coffee" or "I can't give up my pastries and sweets," worried that there would be nothing left to eat to gratify their taste buds or their emotions.

After the outburst and having lost my audience, I changed my approach. In future talks, I would say, "It is true we can't live forever. But if you and your loved ones can extend life 5, 10, or even 20 years and rid the feeling of constantly being sick and running to doctors, what's that worth?"

Nevertheless, I realize that for some people doing the "15 Steps to Health Living" may be unrealistic, overwhelming, or not of interest, even for the sake of family, friends and loved ones. But for those of you who are fully engaged in the quest to change your life and your health, I promise you this book will greatly help you achieve that goal. Let's now start your journey to health.

15 STEPS OF HEALTHY LIVING
PART I
NEW WAY OF THINKING ABOUT HEALTH

Step 1
Starting Your Health Journey

*"Our health always seems much
more valuable after we lose it."*

~ Unknown

In this step, you'll understand:

- The importance of going slowly in making changes.
- Why it's important to focus not on a quick fix but developing a healthy lifestyle.
- How to make changes into a habit.

Your first step on the road to good health is to figure out how you're going to implement this program so it can best work for you. Everyone is in a different place in their journey and will be starting or continuing at a different level. If you have largely embraced a healthy lifestyle but want to use this program for motivation and further information, you may speed through the "15 Steps to Healthy Living." If you do though I believe you will still find much information that feels new or from a different angle.

If you have not led a healthy lifestyle, you will need to implement the steps slowly to allow yourself a gradual transition into healthy living. If you go too quickly, you will feel deprived of that which has heretofore given you pleasure, like eating rich, fatty food and lounging all night on the couch in front of the TV. And you will give up and go back to your old habits.

Lifestyle vs. Quick Fix

For those of you who have a long journey down the healing path, changes may not be immediately dramatic and you may get frustrated with your progress. The way around it is to think of this program not as a quick fix but *a new lifestyle.*

Whether you start and implement 10% or 50% of these new healthy habits, you will be changing your life for the better. Even if you only made a 1% healthy change each month, at the end of the year that's a 12% improvement! *Consistency is better than intensity* when starting anything new. If you're not ready for some of the steps, at least the seed is planted for the future.

Initially I too wanted a quick fix. At first, my motivation for making healthier choices was the short term goal of looking and feeling better and having more energy. I didn't consciously think it would become a lifestyle. But eventually it did. If I ate bad foods or missed a workout, I would start to feel guilty and my body would feel it. At this point, I realized that it's ingrained and an important part of my life.

I'd like that for you. If you miss a workout or skip a nutritious meal, I want you to feel guilty. I want you to make up for it or at the very least have a feeling that you can do better. Such consciousness will fuel you to be proactive in your health choices going forward.

Make Healthy Living a Habit

To make healthy living a lifestyle, you must put in effort and consistency until your healthy living becomes a habit. Research shows this takes at least three weeks, or 21 days on average of practicing the new behavior.

For instance, let's say you replace diet sodas with healthy choices, like vitamin water, coconut water, herbal tea or green tea. After 21 days of doing so, these drinks will now seem like second nature and you may only have an occasional diet soda or give them up altogether. That's a positive health change with only investing 21 days of being consistent and wanting to make a change.

Remember, following a healthy lifestyle is a process, not a destination. That way you can enjoy life along the way.

"If you only care enough for a result,
you'll almost certainly attain it."

~ William James

SUMMING UP

- To succeed, people need to go at their own pace.
- People will start out at different levels of health.
- The way to get around wanting a quick fix is to focus on developing a healthy lifestyle.
- It takes 21 days of consistently doing a behavior for it to become a habit.

Step 2
Healing Comes From Within

"For every drug that benefits a patient, there is a natural substance that can achieve the same effect."
~ Dr. Carl C. Pfeiffer

In this step, you'll learn:

- How the body can heal itself.
- Why meds may be largely unnecessary for many illnesses.
- Ways to fortify your immune system.

If I cut myself, sprain my ankle or burn my hand, does the doctor heal the injury? No. My body heals those injuries. Unfortunately though the prevailing mindset is to look for a quick fix of symptoms. And so we rely on medication for healing.

In most cases, it's unnecessary to do so. Our body has an innate healing power. Take a simple cold or flu. Colds and the flu are caused by viruses invading the body through secretions of the eyes and nose, or through the air. To fight the cold or virus, the body releases white blood cells (lymphocytes) produced by the immune system, which attack and destroy viruses. These same lymphocytes then remember the virus so that the immune system can respond quickly when the same virus attacks again.

The symptoms we experience, like fever, cough, fatigue and congestion are there to help our body heal and constitute what Dr. Geerd Hamer's German New Medicine calls a HEALING CRISIS. For instance, a fever is a way for the body's immune system to dissolve infection, since bacteria are temperature sensitive. Once the symptoms are over, you're well on your way to be fully cured and good as new.

Meds! Meds! Meds!

Unfortunately, conventional medicine views these symptoms and healing cycle as "disease" and something to be eradicated. To do so, your doctor will prescribe medicine which can either delay or stop your natural healing altogether. For instance, you will be advised to take aspirin to lower fever which, unless a fever is dangerously high will interfere with the body's own internal healing mechanism. The body's innate response to heat sensitive viruses or bacteria is to increase the body temperature to dissolve the invading pathogen. Aspirin would counter that mechanism.

Likewise, when you suffer with stomach flu (or food poisoning) and vomit or have diarrhea, your body is ridding and expelling toxins. Taking meds to reduce symptoms is often counter intuitive to normal body function.

HELPFUL TIP: Vomiting and/or diarrhea throws off the body's electrolyte balance. Normally when you sweat from being too hot or working out, you lose electrolytes such as sodium, potassium, chloride, magnesium and calcium. When electrolytes are lost rapidly through vomiting or diarrhea, symptoms may include being irritable, weak, dizzy, sleepy, headache, dry mouth, flushed face, dry warm skin, muscle cramps, lack of urination or urination that is darker than usual. It's vital that these lost fluids are replaced. Drink plenty of water with high quality electrolytes. There are plenty from which to choose. I personally use Ultima Replenisher that contains up to 12 natural electrolytes versus other popular electrolyte sport drinks that may only include three electrolytes and also contain high fructose corn syrup. Another natural source of electrolytes is coconut water. Coconut water contains five key electrolytes. Food sources for electrolytes include bananas, celery, dates, avocados, coconuts, potatoes, olives, tomatoes, kale, spinach and other green leafy vegetables.

Boost Immune System

"Treat the cause not the effect."

~ Dr. Edward Bach

Instead of treating the symptoms of the flu or cold, work to increase your body's ability to fight it. You do this by fortifying your immune system to do the job it was designed to do: combat microorganisms. By eating the right nutrients, being mentally positive and happy, handling stress, exercising and eliminating toxicities you will boost the immune system to allow your body to work optimally and heal itself. Medication will be largely unnecessary except in a life-saving and life sustaining circumstances.

Here is a list of many ways you can enhance your immune system:

1. **Eat fruits and vegetables:** Make sure they're organic.
2. **Eat raw garlic:** Perhaps a bit extreme, but this natural antibiotic increases immunity.
3. **Drink large amounts of fluids:** This will help flush out pathogens.
4. **Exercise:** Moderate exercise stimulates the disease fighting white blood cells in the body to move from the organs to the bloodstream.
5. **Get Chiropractic Adjustments:** There are numerous scientific research studies validating the effectiveness of chiropractic on the immune system (the effects of the adjustments are inextricably linked to the nervous system and immune function).
6. **Get Sufficient Sleep:** You need a good eight hours a night for your body to regenerate and heal.
7. **Relax/Meditate**: Stress has been proven in many research journals to lower your immunity.
8. **Take Supplemental Nutrients**
   - **Vitamin D.** Vitamin D has been getting recent attention in major health journals as a major contributor to building a stronger immune system, especially when not getting enough sun exposure.

- **Vitamin C.** White blood cells may utilize 4 to 6 times the normal rate of vitamin C during a cold or flu (foods: acreola cherry, citrus fruits).
- **Vitamin E.** Builds a healthier immune system (food: almonds, avocados, spinach, wheat germ oil).
- **Zinc.** In the form of amino acid chelated minerals.
- **Multi-vitamins and Minerals.** Strengthens immunity - think prevention.
- **Herbs:** Astragalus, Echinacea, Golden Seal.
- **Airborne or Emergen-C.** A blend of vitamins and herbs specific to building a stronger immune system.
- **Sterols and Sterolins.** Plant "fats" in fruits, vegetables, seeds, and nuts that increase the function of the immune system.
- **Probiotics (i.e. acidophilus).** The good bacteria that help to detoxify and suppress pathogens and backup the immune system.

In summary, take action steps to assist your body's immune system to fight the invading virus or bacteria versus treating the symptoms.

SUMMING UP

- The body can heal itself if the immune system is strong.
- Meds can interfere with the healing process.
- Work to build up your immune system through healthy eating, exercise, chiropractic adjustments, proper sleep and supplementation.

PART II
HONOR YOUR BODY

Step 3
The Foods You Eat

"Let food be thy medicine and medicine be thy food."
~ Hippocrates.

In this step, you'll learn:

- Why we need to eat like our ancestors.
- Why the standard American diet causes disease.
- The importance of eating largely alkaline food.

A colleague and friend of mine shared with me a story of one of his patients who described him as "New Age" because his shelves were full of supplements, vitamins, enzymes, green (vegetable) powder and many other natural health products. Said my friend to him, "I'm not trying to be New Age, I'm trying to get to the Stone Age!"

I laughed. His comments were so on point. We want to go back to a time when we ate whole organic food that came from the earth's untainted soil containing all the vitamins, minerals, nutrients that our body needs.

The Standard American Diet & Disease

Up until around 120 years ago, people did not die from heart disease, strokes, cancer, and autoimmune diseases (diabetes, M.S., Alzheimer's, Parkinson's). In fact, these diseases were rare. They are "lifestyle" diseases that started when we traded food from the earth for unnatural and processed foods.

Today Americans eat 80% man-made processed food. Food containing unnatural flavoring, preservatives, chemicals and dozens of other food additives to make the food look good or taste good. Such food lacks the nutrition our body needs to function.

Nor does our body know what to do with this artificial or unnatural food. Our digestion system was designed to break down and utilize the foods that earth supplied for us. When we eat unnatural food, we feel sick, put on weight, become fatigued, suffer digestive disturbances, and have trouble sleeping.

In his documentary called *Super Size Me,* Morgan Spurlock conducted a fascinating health experiment. He ate three meals exclusively at McDonalds daily for 30 days. His lifestyle dramatically changed as a result as did his physical and psychological well-being. At the end of the 30 day experiment, he gained 24.5lbs, had a 13% body mass increase, a cholesterol level of 230, and experienced listlessness, headaches, depression, mood swings, sexual dysfunction, chest pains, shortness of breath and fat accumulation in his liver. His specialists begged him to abandon this project. And though he did go to an extreme to make his point, the reality is that Americans do this to a slower degree over a lifetime. We're seeing people prematurely dying at an alarming rate.

What's the best option? Eat foods that were here before 120 years ago before the advent of processed foods.

These Brits did. In an experiment for British TV, nine volunteers camped out for twelve days at the Paignton Zoo in Devon, mimicking foods our prehistoric ancestors likely consumed. Guided by a nutritionist, the volunteers consumed raw fruit, vegetables, nuts and honey. On the second week, cooked fish was added. Over twelve days, the average volunteer lost almost 10 pounds, had a 23 percent drop in their cholesterol levels, and their average blood pressure fell from 140/83 (marginally high blood pressure) to 122/76.

Making simple changes can drastically add life and quality of years.

Alkaline/Acid Balance

Our body as you know tries to maintain a constant temperature 98.5F or 37C. It's called homeostasis. But even more, our body works to maintain homeostasis through the right amount of oxygen in our blood, a pH of 7.365, which is slightly alkaline. The higher the pH reading, the more alkaline and oxygen rich the fluid is. Our body is in its healthiest state and flourishes with an alkaline pH.

When our pH is more acidic than alkaline, our blood cannot absorb enough oxygen and our body's organs and fluids don't operate well. This sets up an environment making the human body more susceptible to sickness and disease. As a result of an acidic pH, we feel tired, get depressed, gain weight, and have poor digestion. Eventually, an acidic pH can lead to candida infections, arthritis, diabetes, heart disease or cancer.

Acidic Food

Overacidity happens primarily from eating acidic foods. Acidic foods include meat, poultry, dairy and cheese products, eggs, sugar and refined foods, excess fatty and rich foods, and coffee, tea and alcohol – the typical Standard American Diet (SAD).

These foods increase the transit time of food through the digestive tract and vitamins and minerals might not adequately be assimilated. The worst offender is meat which stays in the body for at least three days, producing much acid waste.

Here's a list of acidic foods which, unfortunately are those that most of us *like most*:

- Junk & processed foods
- Sugar
- All animal food (meat, eggs, chicken, fish, lobster, oysters)
- Grains: white wheat, rice, pasta, flour, bread etc.
- Dairy products (milk, cheese, butter)
- Bad saturated fats (baked goods made with vegetable and canola oil, etc.)
- Peanuts, cashews

Alkaline Foods

The most alkalizing foods are raw green leafy vegetables, non-sweet fruits and wheat grasses. The following is a list of alkaline foods and drinks that help our body to heal itself from most diseases:

- Vegetables - especially raw green leafy vegetables

- Fresh herbs and spices - parsley, basil, cilantro, cayenne, ginger
- Fruits - watermelon, avocado, young coconuts
- Wheatgrass
- Sprouts: sunflower, pea, buckwheat, alfalfa, mung bean, broccoli etc.

The following are the best alkaline drinks.
- Alkaline water
- Coconut water (Young coconut water even better)
- Vegetable juice
- Wheatgrass juice

How Acidic Are You?

How do you know your body's pH? You buy some pH test strips (litmus paper) at a health store and pee on it. The paper will tell you instantly what your pH is and thus, how alkaline or acid you are.

SUMMING UP

- Eat whole, natural food.
- Eat largely alkaline food to optimize your health potential.
- Test your pH with a goal of reaching a morning urine pH between 6.5 and 7.5

STEP 4
Your New Grocery List for
Healthy Weight & Longevity

"Don't eat anything your great-great grandmother wouldn't recognize as food."

~ Michael Pollan

In this step, you'll understand:

- The value of eating real food.
- What are healthy carbs, fats and proteins?
- Why it's important to read food labels on any product.
- Why organic food is best.
- Healthy eating and shopping tips.

For thousands of years, human beings ate nothing but what the earth supplied -- organically grown fruits, vegetables, seeds, nuts and meat. And then in 1903, hydrogenation entered the picture. Hydrogenation is a process to preserve food. Today, 90% of the foods sold in America are processed with chemicals, antibiotics, hormones, food coloring, artificial sugar and other dangerous non-foods.

Does it matter? You bet. Our digestive system was designed to digest the foods available from the earth. Processed foods don't break down properly, robbing us of needed nutrients and making us prone to every imaginable disease. Consider this. At the start of the 20th century, cancer, heart disease and autoimmune disease were rare. People died mostly of infectious disease.

Food is your medicine; food is your poison. If you want to live a long, healthy life, you must revamp your grocery list to food as medicine.

Here's how.

CARBS, FATS & PROTEIN
Carbs

Carbs have gotten a bad reputation of late and low carb diets are all the rage, especially if you want to watch your weight. But is this true? It depends on whether you're talking about good or bad carbs.

Good Carbs

Complex carbs, namely plant foods - vegetables and fruits – deliver the fiber, vitamins, minerals, phytochemicals and antioxidants that your body needs to thrive and feed your brain the fuel it needs to function. Generally found in high fiber food, they break down slowly into your bloodstream and provide a steady blood sugar level through the day. This slow process means that you don't feel hungry and irritable, and especially when that mid-afternoon slump rolls around.

LOADING UP ON GOOD CARBS

For optimal health, load up on the following good carbs.

- Fresh fruit
- Non-starchy vegetables (carrots, celery, cucumber, spinach)
- Starchy root vegetables in moderations (squash, potatoes)
- Cruciferous vegetables (broccoli, cauliflower, kale, peas)
- Nightshade plants in moderation (green pepper, eggplant, tomato)
- Not-gluten grains like buckwheat, millet, quinoa, brown rice, basmati and jasmine rice
- Nuts
- Legumes like beans, alfalfa, peas, chickpeas, lentils, soybeans
- Non-pasteurized dairy products

Bad Carbs

Simple carbohydrates like refined grains (white bread, white rice, white enriched pasta), processed foods (cake, candy, cookies, chips), white potatoes, sweetened soft drinks and SUGAR are bad for you. These bad carbs break down quickly in your bloodstream and flood it with simple sugars (glucose). This quick release causes a surge in the hormone insulin; your blood sugar spikes and you feel edgy. In no time your hand is back in the cookie jar for another quick fix.

And the pattern keeps repeating because your brain gets addicted to the high glucose levels. You crave more and more to keep from feeling down and irritable.

Even worse, too much blood sugar and insulin for too long creates more fat storage, less fat burning, and malfunctioning proteins that can eventually lead to organ damage, adult onset diabetes and even cancer.

WEANING OFF BAD CARBS

If you're addicted to simple carbs, as most Americans are who eat the Standard American Diet (SAD), it will take time to wean yourself off the carb wagon. These simple tips will help free you from their dangerous hold:

Tip 1: Eat Natural Food

Don't buy foods with corn syrup and non-natural colorings, or things that sound like chemicals or artificial fillers. Many store-bought foods and snacks that claim to be 100% natural are not. The Food and Drug Administration does not define natural, so food labels can be misleading.

Tip 2: Eat according to the Glycemic index (GI)

If you're not sure what foods to eat to control blood sugar, follow the Glycemic Index (GI). The GI ranks carbohydrates according to how fast and how far blood sugar rises after eating a food containing carbohydrates and other nutrients. For example, white bread and short grained white rice convert almost immediately to blood sugar that results in a rapid spike. They are high on the GI index. Brown rice, in contrast has a lower GI index as it digests more slowly, causing a lower and gentler shift in blood sugar.

Glycemic Index (GI) for Assorted Foods					
Low		Moderate		High	
Food	GI	Food	GI	Food	GI
Peanuts	14	Apple juice	40	Life Savers	70
Plain yogurt	14	Snickers	41	White bread	70
Soy beans	18	Peach	42	Bagel	72
Peas	22	Carrots	47	Watermelon	72
Cherries	22	Brown rice	50	Popcorn	72
Barley	25	Strawberry jam	51	Graham crackers	74
Grapefruit	25	Power Bar	53	French fries	75
Link sausage	28	Orange juice	53	Grape-Nuts	75
Black beans	30	Honey	55	Shredded wheat	75
Lentils	30	Pita bread	57	Gatorade	78
Skim milk	32	Oatmeal plain	58	Corn flakes	81
Fettuccine	32	Pineapple	59	Rice cakes	82
Chickpeas	33	Sweet potato	61	Pretzels	83
Chocolate milk	32	Coca Cola	63	Baked white potato	85
Whole-wheat spaghetti	37	Raisins	64	Instant rice	87
Apple	38	Cantaloupe	65	Gluten-free bread	90
Pinto beans	39	Whole-wheat bread	67	Dates	103

Tip 3: Choose Rainbow Diet

When choosing your daily fruits and vegetables think the colors of the rainbow and fill your salad plate with varying colors. The more color, the higher the phytonutrients. "Phyto" refers to the Greek word for plant. Phytonutrients or phytochemicals provide health-protecting, antioxidant and anti-inflammatory properties by working synergistically with the vitamins, minerals, and fiber present in fruits and vegetables. Examples of phytonutrients are resveratrol found in red wine and grapes, beta-carotene found in carrots and lycopene found in tomatoes. The deeper the color, the more the phytonutrients.

Tip 4: Let Fiber Be Your Guide

The secret for a carb being good or bad is fiber. Also known as roughage or bulk, fiber is the part of the plant that our body does not digest or absorb. Fiber helps lower blood sugar, slow absorption of sugar into the blood, cut cholesterol, feel full to promote weight control and even eliminate constipation and hemorrhoids.

Whole plant foods and especially fruits, vegetables and beans are very high in fiber. Food made with white flour or white sugar is highly processed and stripped of beneficial fiber.

The recommended amount of daily fiber for the average man or woman is 25 grams, the amount in around three servings each of fruits and vegetables. So make a large salad as your main meal! Another way to get loads of fiber into your diet is to add a few tablespoons of coconut oil to smoothies, baked goods, soups, and hot cereal. And drink fresh coconut water.

Tip 5: Use Natural Sweeteners & Drinks

If you're used to satisfying your taste buds with cookies, cakes, candy, and sodas, one of the toughest challenges for you will be to break this sugar addiction. But you can, though it might take time.

Here are delicious healthier alternatives to processed sugar:

- Naturally-sweetened herbal teas
- Fresh fruit and vegetable juice
- Coconut water
- Honey

- Unrefined maple syrup
- Brown rice syrup
- Coconut aminos

Tip 6: Read Labels

Many of us will eat food without reading labels and actually knowing what it contains. This is a bad way to take charge of your health. The significance of looking at your food labels cannot be over-emphasized. For instance, products that claim to have no sugar added may use carbohydrates such as maltodextrin. Maltodextrin has a glycemic index of 140-150 whereas sugar is 90! Read labels! Here's what to look for:

Total Carbohydrate. Total amount of carbohydrate per serving. Often the grams of "fiber," grams of "sugars" and grams of "other carbohydrate" will add up to the grams of "total carbohydrate" on the label. The daily recommended consumption of carbohydrates is between 45 to 65 percent of your total daily calories.

Dietary Fiber. Total amount of fiber per serving. The daily recommended consumption of fiber is 25 grams.

Sugars. Total amount of carbohydrate from sugar from all sources -- natural sources like lactose and fructose as well as added sugars like high-fructose corn syrup. The American Heart Association recommends most American women eat to no more than 100 calories of sugar per day (20 grams or 4 teaspoons) and no more than 150 calories per day for men (36 grams or 7 ½ teaspoons).

Ingredient. The higher to the top of the list of ingredients the more sugar in the food. The same holds true for fats and sodium (or product ingredients). The higher to the top, the more contained in the product.

SMART EATING TIP: Avoid diet sodas. They have no nutritional value and contain artificial sweeteners (aspartame, saccharin, sucralose) and synthetic added sugars that are extremely damaging to your health. They also trigger weight gain by triggering insulin, which sends your body into fat storage mode, explains Brooke Alpert, RD, author of *The Sugar Detox.*

Tip 7: Eat Organic

More and more, supermarkets are carrying organic food. There's good reason for this: organic food is healthier. Organic fruits and vegetables are grown without dangerous insecticides, herbicides or other chemicals. In other words, it's the food our great-great grandparents grew in their gardens. And research has found organic to taste better.

SMART HEALTH INFO: Eat organic tomatoes! Tomatoes contain more health-protective antioxidants because the absence of pesticides mean none of their nutrients are leached away as a result of the application of harmful chemicals.

What is the difference between all natural food and organic?

Food labeled organic by the USDA is certified to be organic meaning it is guaranteed to not contain toxic synthetic pesticides, toxic synthetic herbicides, or chemical NPK fertilizers used in production, and no antibiotics or growth hormones are given to animals. Look for the USDA Organic Seal. Local farmers who sell organic products in their local communities or at farmers markets are held to the same standards. Ask if their products are either naturally organic certified by the USDA or Certified Naturally Grown (CNG). Food labeled simply as "natural" is not regulated and may contain processed ingredients.

If you cannot always eat organic, eat food with the least amount of pesticides, the toxic substance used to kill weeds, insects, fungus, rodents, etc.

According to the Environmental Working Group, these are the foods with the most amount of pesticides, and should be replaced with organic sources. They are in order from most pesticides used to least used. (https://www.ewg.org/foodnews/dirty_dozen_list.php)

DIRTY DOZEN

1. Strawberries
2. Spinach
3. Nectarines
4. Apples
5. Peaches
6. Pears
7. Cherries
8. Grapes
9. Celery
10. Tomatoes
11. Sweet Bell Peppers
12. Potatoes

Fat

Fats, some experts will tell you, cause excessive weight gain and disease. And this leads some people to buy into a low fat diet.

But are fats *really* bad for you? Absolutely not. Unsaturated high quality fat is necessary to boost thinking, memory, learning and happiness as your brain is about 60 percent fat. Lack of good fat, mostly omega 3s, can lead to depression, poor memory and concentration, anxiety and other mental health issues as can consuming too much bad fat.

Bad Fats = Saturated Fats or Trans Fats (trans fatty acid)

What's bad are hydrogenated or man-made fats, like corn, soy, safflower, and sunflower oils, also called trans fats. Hydrogenation takes liquid unsaturated oils and converts them to solids. This method is used to preserve food so it doesn't go rancid and also to add to a longer shelf life. And while this seems like it would be a good thing, in fact it creates unhealthy trans fats that raise your bad cholesterol (LDL) and lower your good cholesterol levels (HDL). These bad fats also increase your risk of developing heart disease and stroke, as well as developing diabetes.

To reduce trans fats in your diet, the American Heart Association recommends cutting back on foods containing partially hydrogenated vegetable oils. These can include:

- Coffee creamer
- Crackers, cookies, cakes, frozen pies, and other baked goods
- Fast food
- Frozen pizza
- Ready-to-use frostings
- Refrigerated dough products (such as biscuits and cinnamon rolls)
- Snack foods (such as microwave popcorn)
- Vegetable shortenings and stick margarines
- Fried foods

Do your best to avoid eating foods with trans fats by checking labels. Trans fats are listed alongside of saturated fats and cholesterol.

SMART EATING TIP: Though a saturated fat, coconut oil is digested and processed differently than other fats and very healthy. This is because coconut oil makes energy in the body rather than store it as body fat.

Good Fats = Unsaturated Fats

Unsaturated fats like olive and flax are not only very good for you but absolutely essential for brain health. A concentrated source of energy and necessary for proper nerve activity, vitamin absorption, immune system function and healthy cells these good fats lower bad cholesterol in the blood, decrease risk of heart attack, reduce inflammation, stimulate metabolism, and support brain development.

SMART EATING TIP: **When eating out.** Many fast food and chain restaurants will have the nutritional information readily available. If not, ask the server which fats are used for cooking and preparation.

Omega 3's

Essential Fatty Acids, especially omega 3's, are essential for healthy physical and mental wellbeing, normal growth and development and for reducing inflammation and inflammatory conditions. Inadequacy leads to cardiovascular, digestive and immune problems, along with allergies, diabetes, depression, memory problems and foggy thinking.

FASCINATING FACTS: Interestingly, the American Eskimo lived primarily on seal and whale blubber rich in omega 3 fatty acids and cardiovascular disease was all but unheard of.

Omega 3's are found primarily in fatty fish, walnuts and flaxseed oil. As these foods are typically inadequate in the standard American diet, many of us are not getting adequate daily essential fatty acids. Children especially suffer from inadequate omega 3. In a study from Purdue University conducted by Dr. John Burgess, children low in omega 3's were found to be more likely to be hyperactive, develop learning disabilities and exhibit behavioral problems.

I do a lot of presentations on healthy living and always highly recommend Omega 3 supplements. A former patient of mine who attended one of my presentations put her two sons on omega 3 supplementation, both of whom were having attention issues. She raved about how much better they paid attention in school and happily saw health changes, including improved skin complexion.

Getting Daily Essential Fatty Acids

The human body does not generate Omega 3's. They must be obtained through dietary intake from the following, or supplementing.

Plant Oils

Olive (cold-pressed, extra-virgin) is the healthiest, while flaxseed oil is also a major source of omega 3 fatty acids.

Nuts

Walnuts contain high amounts of omega 3's and have high antioxidant activity.

Fatty Fish

Fatty fish is another source of omega 3 fatty acids. Salmon, mackerel, sardines and herring are the types of fish highest in this essential fat and, if wild, are lower in mercury than other fish. Nevertheless, all fish have mercury because of the polluting of our ocean, lake and river waters and, as mercury is toxic for human consumption I encourage an omega 3 supplement over eating fish.

SMART EATING TIP: To get more beneficial omega 3 fatty acids, add flax, hemp, chia, and walnuts to your diet. Try throwing them into your morning smoothie.

Proteins

To have strength and energy, our body needs protein for building tissue and for growth and repair of muscles. You can get quality protein both from animal sources and from non-animal sources.

Animal Sources for Protein

- Free-range chickens
- Grass-fed beef
- Organic turkey
- Seafood
- Unpasteurized Milk, Cheese, and Yogurt
- Organic Eggs

SMART EATING TIP: To avoid toxins, hormones, antibiotics and other harmful substances, eat free range, organic and preferably grass-fed beef, eggs and poultry. Avoid at all costs processed meat and cold cuts, bacon, sausages, hot dogs and barbecued meat. They contain chemicals toxic to your health.

Non-Flesh & Non-Animal Protein Sources

- Quinoa
- Beans
- Tempeh, a fermented soy product
- Nuts & Seeds
- Sprouts, particularly sunflower and pea sprouts

Genetically Modified Organisms (GMO's)?

GMO's, also referred to as Genetically Engineered Foods, Genetic Engineering, Genetically Modified, Genetically Modified Seeds are foods created by taking genetic material (DNA) from one species (plant, seeds, animal, bacteria, or virus) and transferring it to another species to create a combinations of genes. According to the World Health Organization this process alters genetic material (DNA) in a way that does not occur naturally.

Some of the most common foods that are genetically modified include livestock, corn, soy, corn starch, vegetable oils, sugar beets, and many of the food products intended for children, in which parents give their kids daily.

Are these foods safe for human consumption? This is a controversy because the effect of long-term consumption are unknown. For this reason, scientists from the FDA have warned of allergies, toxins, new diseases, mutations, cancers and nutritional problems and urged long term studies. Most health, wellness and longevity experts adamantly oppose eating GMO's, myself included.

FYI: While most developed nations require GMO foods to be labeled, and some have restricted or banned GMO's, the US has neither labeled them nor restricts their consumption.

How can you protect yourself from consuming GMO's? Eat organic as much as possible. Look for non-GMO's and avoid ingredients such as corn, soy, canola, sugar beets, high fructose corn syrup, maltodextrin, soy protein to name a few.

Gluten

Gluten is a form of a protein found in wheat and other related grains such as barley, rye, and oat. Some of the most common foods with gluten are breads, pastas, crackers, seasonings, and spice mixes.

Most of us eat these foods daily. This is a problem. Gluten is difficult to break down and digest.

Gluten Intolerance

Gluten is especially difficult to digest for those with gluten intolerance, a condition that has sky rocketed in recent years. Symptoms range from mild to severe and include diarrhea, fatigue, weight loss, skin rash, brain fog, bloating, gas, and other digestive discomfort.

Celiac Disease

More serious than gluten intolerance is Celiac disease, an autoimmune disorder in which your immune system attacks the gluten. Common symptoms of celiac disease include the same symptoms as above, but more severe.

Cause

The cause of gluten intolerance is unknown but scientists speculate it's from either the processing or the way the wheat was grown.

How to know if you have a sensitivity

Your physician can give you a blood test to assess if the antibodies associated with gluten intolerance are present. Or you can just eliminate gluten in your diet and see if your symptoms subside or go away.

Going Gluten Free

Here's a few tips on how to go gluten free:

Tip 1: Eat gluten-free grains such as buckwheat, quinoa, chia, flax, beans, legumes, millet, rice and potatoes.

Tip 2: Use gluten-free flours such as almond flour or coconut flour.

Tip 3: Avoid processed fruits, vegetables and lean meats which may contain gluten.

Eat to Increase Metabolism

Metabolism slows as we age and you know what that means: weight gain. A few years ago, I put together, along with a former patient who is a teacher, an informal survey to assess school aged children's perception on health. To my shock, most kids associate weight gain and developing diseases as part of normal aging. It's not. Though time works against us, weight gain and disease are not inevitable if you are proactive in your health. Here are some ways to boost your metabolism with minimal effort:

Tip 1: Eat metabolism boosting foods like almonds, beans, berries, cinnamon, coconut oil, apple cider vinegar, chia seeds, and spinach. They will help you speed up your metabolism so you have more energy, feel firmer, lose weight more easily and even sleep better.

Tip 2: Eat so you're not hungry but not until you feel full. Use smaller plates to encourage smaller portions versus larger plates that encourage larger portions.

Tip 3: Eat four to five smaller meals throughout the day and two healthy snacks to maintain sugar level.

FYI: Metabolism works like a camp fire: the fire is your metabolism and the logs are your meals. If you add smaller logs more often, the better the fire while large logs will slow the fire and may smother it. Stick with the smaller logs (meals) more often to keep an efficient burning campfire (metabolism).

Tip 4: Eat breakfast to jump-start metabolism. After sleeping 7-9 hours, the body needs to fuel a strong metabolism.

Tip 5: Drink a cup of brewed tea which can raise your metabolism by 12%, according to one Japanese study. This is likely due to the antioxidant catechins in tea.

Tip 6: Remember to eat high fiber foods to help you burn fat better.

Tip 7: Eat organic as toxins interfere with the energy-burning process.

Tip 8: Include protein in every meal as the body needs protein to maintain lean muscle. Also, research shows that protein increases post-meal calorie burn by as much as 35%.

Tip 9: Women, especially pre-menopausal need to get enough iron in their diets. Iron is essential for carrying to your muscles the oxygen needed to burn fat. Excellent sources include shellfish, lean meats, beans, fortified cereals, and spinach.

Tip 10: Get out in the sun as vitamin D is essential for preserving metabolism-revving muscle tissue. Most doctor's offices now test for vitamin D to see if your levels are adequate.

Tip 11: Add Organic Apple Cider Vinegar to your diet. Though it may not directly increase metabolism, it may help to burn and regulate blood sugar which indirectly influences metabolism.

Tip 12: Follow my favorite way to influence metabolism by choosing how much and when to eat carbohydrates (needed for energy); proteins (needed for healing, building and repairing the body); and fats (needed for cell structure, brain and organ function, as well hormone production):

Morning meal(s): Eat high to moderate amounts of carbohydrates, low protein and low fat. After sleeping for 7 to 9 hours, your body needs energy from healthy carbs to get going.

One of my favorite breakfast dishes is a bowl of oatmeal with rice milk sprinkled with raw almonds, flax seeds and blueberries.

Midday meal(s): Eat moderate carbohydrates, protein and fat.

Evening meal(s): Eat low carbohydrates, high protein and moderate to high fat. In the evening, when your body is getting ready to sleep it doesn't need carbs for energy. It needs protein for healing, building and repair while sleeping, along with moderate to high fats.

A good evening meal might be lean chicken or fatty fish like salmon and organic vegetables, or a kale salad with coconut oil. A bowl of spaghetti in contrast will result in weight gain because carbohydrates or unused energy will be stored as fat.

Drink Water

Staying hydrated is critical to regulate all body functions, including metabolic reactions, cellular function, digestion, temperature regulation, transportation of nutrients and removal of waste. This is because the average adult's body composition is 65% to 70% water (varies with age, sex, health and weight).

Water composition results from the foods you eat (fruits, vegetables, etc.), the water you drink, and to a much lesser extent liquids like coffee, juices, milk, and so on. As the average person eats little raw vegetables and fruits and is not in the habit of drinking water frequently, most people are chronically dehydrated. Yet few people are unaware that they are because they mistake thirst for hunger.

Could you be a victim of dehydration? You likely are if you get tired easily as dehydration is the number one trigger of daytime fatigue.

How to Stay Hydrated

There's an easy solution to dehydration: drink a clean water supply daily of filtered water to equal half your body weight (128 pounds equals 8 glasses of water, or 64 ounces). This step is one of the easiest ways to help your body become healthier.

Side Bar: Why filtered water versus tap water? An Associated Press investigation found pharmaceuticals including antibiotics, hormones, mood stabilizers and other medication found in the water supply in 24 major cities in the U.S. Another study shows dangerous chemicals such as chlorine, fluoride, lead, as well as farm and industrial contaminants, have also been found in our water supply.

Many grocery stores now have a 5-phase filtration process built into their self-service water refilling area. Drinking clean filtered water is an important step in optimizing your health.

5-phase Filtration

1. Activated Carbon Filter to remove chlorine and odors.

2. Micron Filter to remove dirt, rust and other particles.

3. Reverse Osmosis to remove salts and impurities.

4. Post carbon filter improves taste of water.

5. Ultraviolet light to ensure safe, high quality water.

Grocery stores that offer this service also have reusable plastic 3 to 5 gallon containers available that are usually BPA (bisphenol A) free. An industrial chemical made in plastics, BPA is hazardous to your health and can leach into water and even food if you're using BPA plastics as containers. If you're not sure, look for the BPA free label or imprint usually on the bottom of the container and/or bottle. All your drinking containers, including drinking bottles and food containers, should have the BPA free label. If not, I'd recommend switching them out to BPA free immediately.

Don't Overdo Salt

Watch your salt intake. Processed salt lacks the full spectrum of minerals and other nutrients that protect and enhance your health and can cause high blood pressure and other health problems. Use natural salt instead like Himalayan salt which contains 84 minerals and trace minerals, including iodine.

SIDE BAR: **Try the 60-day diet modification to help reduce the symptoms of allergies**

If you're struggling with allergies, try the following steps to help your immune system combat sensitivities to allergens.

- **No Dairy Products:** no milk, cheese, butter, mayonnaise, alfredo sauce, yogurt, ice cream, dairy-based salad dressings
- **No Gluten:** no gluten containing products such as wheat bread, pizza, pasta, cookies, cakes
- **No White Sugar**: read labels as sugar is added to many foods beyond candy, cookies and cakes.

Healthy Eating Tips

- **Eat sitting down in a quiet, relaxed atmosphere.** Turn off the TV or computer as this will cause you to eat unconsciously and possibly overeat.
- **Eat slowly and chew your food thoroughly.** Take time to taste your food and savor the textures and tastes. This is what the French are famous for and we all know the reputation of French cuisine.
- **Drink sparingly with your meals.** Too much liquid will dilute stomach acid and digestive enzymes and you won't digest your food well.
- **Eat when relaxed.** If you are tired, upset or stressed, your sympathetic nervous system takes over and blood gets shunted away from the stomach to the muscles. Also, when stressed, you are more likely to binge on unhealthy comfort foods and drinks. The next time

you're under such distress, plant a mental seed to prep and avoid such splurging.

- **Chew slowly.** This will partially predigest the food in your mouth to help you better digest and assimilate your food. Chewing helps release enzymes in the saliva that break down food further for nutrient absorption. Chewing also signals the start of other digestive processes along the digestive tract.
- **Eat your heaviest meal early in the day.** Avoid eating three to four hours before going to bed to give your digestion a rest. This will help your system rebuild during sleep.
- **Eat small meals frequently throughout the day.** This helps to keep blood sugar levels steady. Eat only when hungry.

Shopping Tips

- Avoid shopping when hungry.
- Shop in the outer aisles, where the fresh food is located.
- Read labels.
- Don't shop when in a hurry.
- Shop with a list and stick to it.

SUMMING UP

HEALTHY CARBS, FATS & PROTEINS
CARBS

- To get healthy carbs, eat fresh, preferably organic vegetables, moderate amount of starchy & anti-oxidizing vegetables and fresh, preferably organic fruits and beans

- Eat according to Glycemic Index (GI)
- Choose a rainbow diet
- Use natural sweeteners
- Drink natural drinks like herbal tea and coconut water

FATS

To get healthy fats, eat healthy omega 6's, such as seeds and nuts and load up on omega-3 EFA (Essential Fatty Acid).

PROTEINS

Get healthy protein from both animals and non-flesh food.

- Flesh (Animal Sources)
  - o Poultry
  - o Lean Beef
  - o Seafood
  - o Unpasteurized Milk, Cheese, and Yogurt
  - o Eggs
- Non-Flesh (Vegetarian Sources)
  - o Beans
  - o Tempeh, a fermented soy product
  - o Sprouts, particularly sunflower and pea sprouts
- Load your diet with enough fiber
- Read labels
- Eat organic
- Stay hydrated
- Eat to increase metabolism
- Watch the salt

Step 5
Healthy Digestion

In this chapter, you'll understand:

- The importance of healthy digestion.
- Why it is necessary to take enzyme supplements.
- Why it is essential to fill your gut with good bacteria from probiotics and fermented food and drinks.

"All disease begins in the gut." So said Hippocrates about 2400 years ago. If you wish to be healthy you must have healthy digestion. To do so requires getting enough enzymes to digest your food and having a strong microbiome or good gut flora.

Get Enough Enzymes

Enzymes, gotten largely from fruits and vegetables, are necessary to help us digest the food we eat and break it down to useable, absorbable nutrients. Yet, the average American's body is depleted of enzymes. There are three reasons for this depletion:

1. We eat little fresh fruits and vegetables.
2. We cook most of our food and enzymes are destroyed at temperatures of 118° F. or above.
3. As we grow older, we also lose our ability to produce concentrated digestive enzymes and therefore do not digest our food as well.

How do you know if you're enzyme deficient? Your body will react with "indigestion," like burping, heartburn, abdominal pain, bad breath, excess gas, skin problems, diarrhea and constipation. In addition, your body may react with headaches, mental fatigue, nervousness, lack of concentration, memory loss, insomnia, all as a result from not having enzymes.

To replenish enzymes, consume daily these enzyme rich foods.

- Raw, organic fruits and vegetables
- Sprouts
- Chlorophyll rich greens
- Fermented foods

To further aid digestion, it's a good idea to take digestive enzyme supplements just prior to or with your meals.

Reestablish Gut Flora

The healthy gut contains over 100 trillion microorganisms from some 400 different species. This good bacteria eats up bad bacteria to help you digest your food and keep your immune system strong. But if you eat processed food and take medication for every ailment, this balance is upset and your gut likely contains more harmful, putrefying bacteria. Further common dietary and lifestyle factors destroy these bacteria such as stress, carbonated drinks, lack of sleep, laxatives and birth control pills, antibacterial herbs and cortisone.

When depleted of bowel flora or good bacteria, the body is prone to numerous diseases including colitis, diabetes, meningitis, rheumatoid arthritis, thyroid disease and even bowel cancer. Even the common cold and the flu are more frequent and debilitating.

Especially problematic is the overuse of antibiotics. Antibiotics not only kill the bad bacteria they also wipe out the good strain of bacteria. So, while you take antibiotics for your cold or ear infection, you may be letting other potential inflammatory conditions go unchecked leading to other problems.

Fortunately, you can greatly increase the good bacteria in your gut by taking probiotics. In fact, the Greek meaning of "probiotics" means "for life."

Getting Probiotics into Your Diet

There are two ways to get probiotics into your diet: eating cultured and fermented food and taking a probiotic supplement. The first way will confer many more probiotics than you will get from supplements.

Fermented Food

- Cultured vegetables such as sauerkraut, beets and pickles
- Cultured dairy, such as yogurt and kefir
- Tempeh and miso
- Kombucha tea
- Kimchi
- Manuka honey

Food Preparation

We have many choices in preparing our food. The following methods are listed from to best to worst.

Raw (preferred)

Fruits and vegetables, sprouted grains, unroasted nuts and seeds, seaweed or beans in the rawest "alive" state is the healthiest form for human absorption. Food preparation below 118° F is the baseline for optimal consumption as food heated above 118° F breaks down the nutrients and natural enzymes and makes digestion more difficult. For the most part, anything outside the produce isle is not in a raw state.

Strive to eat between 50-75% uncooked "alive" raw foods daily. A good way to accomplish this is to make a hefty salad the main meal and everything else side dishes. Include a rainbow variety of colors.

WELLNESS TIP: Many wellness experts encourage those battling illnesses to eat raw foods. This is because raw foods take less metabolic processes for the body to absorb and digest and this allows more of the body's internal metabolic resources to fight the illness.

Steaming

Steaming works by using the steam from boiling water to heat foods. Of all the cooking methods for vegetables, this works best to keep taste and nutrients intact.

Boiling

While commonly used to prepare vegetables, doing so at high temperatures over time can cause a significant loss of nutrients. To help reduce nutritional loss and keep more nutrients in the food, keep the boil to a simmer, or, even better steam your vegetables.

SMART EATING TIP: Keep the vitamin rich water from steaming and boiling to make home-made soups.

Broiling/Grilling

Broiling is heat from a directed heat source coming from top-down; grilling is from a source from the bottom-up, typically using heated coals, wood or gas. Both are commonly used to heat meats quickly but this is not a healthy way of cooking as cooking meats too quickly can cause HCAs (heterocyclic amines), which are cancer causing chemicals.

Here are some ways to reduce the amount of HCA's using these cooking methods: reduce cooking time in the extreme heat; avoid direct open flame cooking; continually turn the meat and remove the charred portion before consuming. Also, broiling is healthier than grilling because it allows fatty grease to drip, reducing saturated fat from the red meat.

INTERESTING FACT: Grilled sea foods have less HCA's and grilled fruits or vegetable don't produce HCA's.

Baking/Roasting – Both are dry-heat cooking methods using temperatures of 300 degrees Fahrenheit or higher. They are an unhealthy way to prepare food because they destroy heat-sensitive vitamins and enzymes and produce trans fats. Using coconut oil and olive oil will reduce the formation of trans fats.

Sautéing – This method of cooking uses a small amount of healthy cooking oil, such as extra-virgin olive oil, in a shallow pan under high heat. To maintain as many nutrients as possible, stir frequently and sauté minimally (3 to 5 minutes) or when the vegetables, meat or fish are tender and avoid burning.

Frying (avoid) – Frying or deep frying oils and fats is highly undesirable as it leads to eating unhealthy fats and high calories. Further, eating fried foods regularly can increase your chance of developing obesity, diabetes, cardiovascular disease, including strokes, and even cancer.

Microwave (avoid) – Microwave cooking is perhaps the most used cooking method and the worst choice. Personally I have never owned a microwave oven and have never used microwave cooking for the following reasons.

1. Microwave ovens use microwaves, a form of an electromagnetic field (EMF) that changes the structure of the molecule. This can degrade nutrients as Hans Hertel, a Swiss chemist discovered. Using blood samples, he also found increased cholesterol levels, decreased hemoglobin (creating anemic tendencies), decreased lymphocyte (white blood cell), and marked increase in leukocytes which are necessary for an immune response to foreign bodies.

IMPORTANT FINDINGS: A study in *The Lancet* showed ten minutes of microwaved infant formula altered the structure of its amino acids, possibly resulting in structural, functional and immunological (immune) abnormalities.

2. Microwave ovens leak radiation. In fact, the FDA even provides a warning to minimize radiation exposure

from new microwave ovens. They recommend that you look at your oven carefully, and not use an oven if the door doesn't close firmly or is bent, warped, or otherwise damaged.

Nevertheless current FDA guidelines permit a certain degree of radiation leakage, though continued use over time may damage human cells and tissues and contribute or lead to cancer.

INTERESTING FACT: Russia recognized dangers in microwave cooking and banned microwave ovens in 1976.

Safe Cookware/Bakeware and Utensils

Look for safe cookware and bakeware products as conventional cookware can be a source of toxins and other harmful materials that can leach into your food. Avoid containers made of aluminum, Teflon or other non-stick coated material. I've found high-grade stainless steel, ceramic, and stoneware good choices. These can be found in most kitchen retail stores.

SUMMING UP

Enzymes

Enzymes are necessary to healthy digestion. Because the standard American diet is largely devoid of enzymes, most of us are enzyme deficient. To compensate, it's necessary to load up on fresh fruits and vegetables and add enzyme supplementation.

Reestablish Gut Flora

The secret to a healthy life is healthy microbiome made up of good bacteria to eat up bad bacteria. This helps you digest your food and keeps your immune system strong. Modern life interferes with the balance of good and bad bacteria in the gut. To compensate, we must take probiotics and load up on fermented food and drinks.

Food Preparation

How you prepare your food and with what are important considerations for optimal health. Raw is the healthiest and steaming is an option for heated vegetables. Also do your homework on the type of cookware, bakeware and utensils to use for the safest preparation.

Step 6
Vitamins & Supplements

"By the proper intakes of vitamins and other nutrients and by following a few other health practices from youth or middle age on, you can, I believe, extend your life and years of well-being by twenty-five to even thirty five years."

~ Linus Pauling

In this chapter, you'll understand:

- We all need to take supplements to maintain good health and longevity.
- Which vitamins and supplements promote good health.
- Why it's best to buy higher priced supplements.

If you eat the whole foods suggested in Step 4, you will go a long way in getting the nutrition you need. Nevertheless, in this day and age of chemicals everywhere, soil depleted of needed minerals, and junk food at every street corner, we can't rely just on our food to get all the nutrition we need. We need to take additional measures, including taking daily supplements.

With 1000's of vitamins to choose from, walking through vitamin shops can be overwhelming. To simplify the task, I have created a list of vitamins and supplements especially advantageous to health and well-being. I personally take all the supplements listed below and at times the additional vitamins listed, as a part of my daily wellness plan for optimal health.

TO BE SAFE: Those under medical care taking medication should consult your health care provider before taking any of these supplements. Some supplements, depending on the brand and/or type may have negative interactions with medication.

WISE ADVICE: For those who have health needs beyond this book, I recommend visiting a reputable alternative or holistic health care provider, naturopath or nutritionist.

Take a Multivitamin

Though you may be healthily, you may unknowingly not be getting all the vitamins and minerals you need in your diet. To insure you do, it's best to add a multivitamin to your daily regimen.

Load up on Omega 3 EFA (Essential Fatty Acid)

In Step 4, the importance Omega 3 was discussed. Let me reiterate: the human body does NOT generate Omega 3, it must be obtained through dietary intake by eating fatty fish, walnuts and flaxseed oil. If you do not eat these foods daily, it's best to supplement.

Enzyme Supplementation

There are many types of enzymes, but the enzymes we're referring to here are digestive enzymes. Digestive enzymes are produced in our body and work in the gastrointestinal tract to help break down foods into smaller and more absorbable material. They help break down protein (protease), carbohydrates (amylase), fats (lipase) and fiber (cellulase). Digestive enzymes in our digestive system become depleted with age, processed and fast food diets, unfiltered water, some medication etc. Signs of depleted enzymes include gas, bloating, abdominal pain, nausea, heartburn, skin problems, mood swings, joint problems and other serious conditions. Digestive enzyme supplementation helps to optimize digestion for nutritional absorption. Another type of enzyme is food enzymes, which are found naturally in raw food and are abundant by eating organic raw fruits and vegetables. These enzymes help start of digestive process.

Probiotic Supplementation
Supplementing with probiotics will insure proper gut flora, proper digestion, proper nutritional absorption and assists with fighting infection and boosting the immune systems. This supplement is known as "good" bacteria and assists in keeping good to bad bacteria balance throughout your gastrointestinal system.

Vitamin D
Produced in your skin in response to sunlight, vitamin D helps regulate the absorption of calcium and phosphorous, facilitates normal immune system function, regulates our mood, counters depression and so much more. Without sufficient vitamin D, normal growth and development of bones and teeth suffer and you have

reduced resistance against certain diseases. Since vitamin D has a factor in the immune system, many studies validate its positive affect on many cancers, as well helping the body fight common cold and flu.

All this makes vitamin D crucial for optimal health and most wellness doctor's visits include vitamin D testing to check for deficiencies. Yet because we spend much more time indoors than out in the sun few of us get sufficient vitamin D and most of the US population is deficient. As such, it's important to supplement vitamin D daily.

Curcumin (or Turmeric) Supplement
Curcumin, widely known as turmeric comes from the ginger family. A powerful tonic for reducing inflammation, it helps speed up healing from tissue and bone injuries and also has skin healing properties. It's also a very strong antioxidant and is being explored for combating several forms of cancer.

Eat Antioxidant Rich Food
We use oxygen to oxidize (burn) food for energy. Called oxidation, this "burning" process results in dangerous free radicals, unstable oxygen atoms that cause damage to neighboring cells and tissues and cause disease. Excessive sun exposure, cigarette smoke, alcohol, saturated fats, pollution and chemicals found in the air and water, fried foods, excessive exercise, and even our own metabolic by-products can all create free radicals, making us sick and prematurely aging us. Antioxidants capture and neutralize free radicals and escort them out of the body before they can cause any additional damage.

Antioxidants include Vitamins A, C, E, beta-carotene, selenium, zinc, magnesium, manganese, and copper.

You can take antioxidants in the form of a Multi-Antioxidant pill that includes all of the antioxidant vitamins listed above in addition to many other common antioxidants used in supplements today.

***SMART HEALTH TIP:* Drink a Glass of Wine.** Resveratrol, a popular antioxidant is a naturally occurring substance derived from the skin of grapes and raspberries, along with some other fruits. Its presence in red and white wine is one of the reasons behind the popular advice that a glass of wine a day is good for your heart and skin and has antidiabetic qualities along with cancer prevention. And it has anti-depressive qualities as well. If you do drink a glass of wine with your meal, make sure it's organic to insure the fruit is grown without artificial or synthetic chemicals, such as herbicides and pesticides. If you're not a wine drinker, resveratrol supplements are available.

***SMART HEALTH TIP:* Have a Green Smoothie for Breakfast.**
Green smoothies consist of blending the combination of fresh leafy greens (kale, spinach, cauliflower, broccoli, romaine, parsley, celery, wheatgrass or algae), fruit (banana, strawberry, mango, pineapple, pomegranate, acai berry or avocado) and a liquid base (filtered water, coconut water, almond milk, rice milk, green tea or organic fruit juices). You can also add coconut oil powder, maca powder, almond butter, yogurt, hemp, chia, or flax seeds. Green smoothies give your body optimal vitamins,

minerals and antioxidants as well as hundreds of phytonutrients that promote optimum health and offer superior and quick (within 30 minutes) absorption and assimilation of nutrients. And in a smoothie, you are getting three times the quantity of greens blended than in a salad and more quickly for those with a busy schedule.

So, have a daily smoothie. For even more nutrition, add green powder mix, spirulina and chlorella.

Green Powder Mix

Green or superfood powder mixes are derived from naturally-occurring foods and give you multiple servings of vegetables, fruits, grasses, algae and other superfoods in a water-soluble scoop. This is a comprehensive way to get vitamins, digestive enzymes, probiotics, herbs and many other health supporting ingredients including spirulina and chlorella.

Spirulina

Spirulina is a blue-green algae with miraculous healing qualities. A "superfood," it is beneficial for heart problems, weight loss, diabetes, metabolic issues, mental disorders, emotional disorders, ADHD, anxiety and depression. Because of its high antioxidant qualities, it's also a cancer preventative. One study showed a 38% regression in cancerous activity resulting from the chewing of betel tree leaf.

Chlorella

Chlorella is single-cell green algae that helps the body detoxify by eliminating unwanted metals and toxins. It helps as well in boosting energy, weight loss, strengthens healthy hormonal function, contributes to cardiovascular health, neutralizes the harmful side-effects of chemotherapy and radiotherapy, decreases blood pressure and lowers cholesterol. We'll discuss more on Chlorella in Step 7 Detoxification.

SMART EATING TIP: For avid exercisers, vegan/vegetarians, or if feel you may not be getting enough protein consider taking whey protein in your smoothie.

SMART EATING TIP: It's healthy to balance fats and carbohydrates with protein in every meal.

The supplements listed to this point I recommend for everyone, which in my opinion will optimize your health and add to your wellbeing. Below are additional supplemental considerations.

Additional Vitamin Considerations

Co-enzyme Q10

Coenzyme Q10 (CoQ10) is part of the makeup of every cell and is necessary to release the energy required for cell regeneration and growth. An antioxidant, it protects against harmful substances within the body. CoQ10 can be found in potent quantity in the meat from organs like the heart and liver. Soy oil, mackerel and sardines also contain high amounts of CoQ10. If you don't routinely eat these foods, it's best to supplement CoQ10.

Acetyl-l-carnitine and Alpha-lipoic acid

Naturally produced by the body, Acetyl-l-carnitine and Alpha-lipoic acid are amino acids essential for metabolism and the release of energy. Both are common dietary supplements immensely helpful for people dealing with consistent fatigue and metabolic problems.

N-Acetyl Cysteine (NAC)

NAC is closely related to and derived from L-cysteine, an essential amino acid in the body. Along with reducing cholesterol levels, NAC substantially reduces the risk of heart diseases. NAC is also an indispensable supplement for people with kidney related problems, since it substantially lowers their risk of a heart attack and stroke.

Glucosamine & Chondroitin Sulfate

In his 1997 New Your Times bestselling book, *The Arthritis Cure,* Dr. Jason Theodosakis shed light on the importance of glucosamine and chondroitin sulfate for joint health. Generally sold and taken together, both have become staple supplements for joint related conditions.

Calcium & Magnesium

Most people are aware of the importance of calcium for strong bones and teeth. But many people are unaware of the importance of magnesium to control muscle aches or spasms, anxiety, poor digestion and trouble sleeping.

If you have poor posture, slouch in front of a computer for hours, have a chronic nagging reoccurring injury, or a physically demanding job or hobby, consider taking calcium and magnesium. Both should be taken together as calcium may not be fully absorbed without magnesium.

BE AWARE: Drinking dark colored soda negatively affects your body's ability to utilize magnesium. Most sodas contain phosphate. Phosphate binds with magnesium in the digestive tract and causes magnesium to be unavailable for your body's utilization. Even drinking soda with a balanced meal can flush magnesium from your body. For those who have a history of osteopenia or osteoporosis ("porous bones"), drinking soda pop should absolutely be avoided.

Which brand(s) of dietary supplements should I purchase?

This question is confusing for many people as so many brands are available in your health store and online. In general, alternative or holistic health care providers or a licensed nutritionist are the best resource for high quality supplements. They will usually recommend and carry products that have been through strict guidelines for manufacturer testing for safety and efficacy.

How do you know if the company has independent organizations testing their products? Go to the company's website. There is usually a manufacturing quality assurance page describing the manufacturing and testing of their products. They may also include it on the label of the product.

In addition to these independent organizations, the U.S government also has standards to ensure quality over supplement manufacturers.

FYI: If you want to research the products you're currently taking or those that you are considering taking, you can use The Dietary Supplement Label Database from the National Institute on Health. This is a database of all dietary supplements currently sold in the U.S. The link is: https://www.dsld.nlm.nih.gov/dsld/

Price

Typically, high quality supplements cost more because they follow the highest standards and quality. This includes testing to ensure that the ingredients break down during the digestive process so the body can utilize the vitamins or minerals (active ingredients).

Years ago, I took an x-ray of a patient to evaluate his spinal condition. Upon closer inspection, I could see small circular outlines at the level of the large intestines. Those circular outlines were undigested vitamins that had passed the digestive process without being absorbed. Obviously, this patient didn't get the any benefit from going with a low-quality and low cost supplement.

SUMMING UP

In this day and age of toxins and dangerous chemicals in our food, air and water, living a long and healthy life requires not just eating healthy food but also taking important nutritional supplements.

These include:

- Multi-Vitamin
- Omega 3
- Enzymes
- Probiotics
- Vitamin D
- Curcumin (or Turmeric)
- Antioxidants and Green Smoothies

Additional Supplements to Consider

- Co-enzyme Q 10

- Acetyl-l-carnitine and Alpha-lipoic acid
- N-Acetyl Cysteine (NAC)
- Glucosamine & Chondroitin Sulfate
- Calcium Magnesium

Buy high quality dietary supplements to insure you're getting what's indicated on the label.

Step 7
Detoxing from Inside

In this chapter, you'll understand:

- The benefits of internal cleansing.
- Why it's important to start with cleansing the colon and then the liver.
- The need to remove heavy metals from the body.
- Why we need to sweat it out.

In this day and age of polluted air, polluted water, polluted food, all our bodies are overly toxic. In fact, research conducted by the Environmental Working Group in collaboration with Commonweal found an average of 200 industrial chemicals and pollutants in the umbilical cord blood of 10 newborn babies studied.

To be healthy, function at your best and live a long life, you must eliminate toxic debris through detoxification. Removing toxins has the following benefits:

1. Preventing chronic disease
2. Enhancing immune system function
3. Losing weight
4. Slowing premature aging
5. Improving quality of life
6. Increasing energy
7. Improving skin quality
8. Boosting mental and emotional clarity

Cleanse Your Colon

The best way to start is to clean out the colon, or large intestine, the "solid waste management" organ in the body. To do so, eat a high fiber diet and flush out debris with herbs, enemas, occasional fasting and, if you wish, a colon cleansing kit.

Here's a suggested occasional cleansing fast plan. Do this fast for one to three days every couple of months.

Before Breakfast:

- 2 ounces wheatgrass juice

Breakfast:

- 16 ounces green drink made from vegetables such as: celery, cucumbers, parsley, kale, watercress, dandelion and sprouts such as sunflower, green pea and fenugreek

Lunch:

- 16 ounces green drink
- Two cups herbal tea

Evening:

- 2 ounces wheatgrass juice

Between-Meal Snacks:

- Lemon water sweetened with stevia or herbal tea

Cleanse Your Liver

After cleansing the colon, it's time to cleanse your liver. This is crucial as the liver's job is to send toxins to the appropriate organ to exit the body. And in today's world, stress, pesticides, food chemicals, environmental toxins, caffeine, nicotine, and prescription, over-the-counter, and recreational drugs greatly tax the liver.

Here's how to detoxify your liver:

- Eat in volume cruciferous vegetables (broccoli, collards, kale, cauliflower, etc.), along with artichokes, asparagus, celery, radishes, cilantro and beets.
- Throw turmeric (curcumin), rosemary and lemon peel (zest instead of just squeezing the lemon juice) into your dishes.
- Consume flaxseeds daily.
- Eat foods containing glutathione such as avocado, asparagus, squash, potato, watermelon, and vegetables like spinach and parsley.
- Eat chlorophyll rich foods like chlorella, spirulina, wheat grass juice or barley juice.
- Take the herb milk thistle.
- Upon awakening, add to a glass of filtered water the juice of 1 lemon, 1 to 2 tablespoons extra-virgin, cold-pressed olive oil, 1 to 2 crushed garlic cloves and a sprinkle of cayenne pepper.

Detoxify Heavy Metals

The next step after cleansing the colon and the liver is to get the heavy metals out of your system. Because we are so exposed to mercury, lead, arsenic and other heavy metals, many of our systems are overloaded with heavy metals. If you feel constantly fatigued, have allergies, skin conditions and autoimmune disorders, it's best to start by having a naturopath or holistic physician test your heavy metal levels. If they're high, you may need a physician to chelate them out of your body.

Nevertheless, there is much you can do daily to reduce your heavy metal load.

Tip 1: Amalgam Removal: Go to a dentist and have your silver amalgam tooth fillings removed, as they are the greatest source of mercury poisoning. A holistic dentist trained in removing amalgam fillings is recommended. Most holistic dentists recommended a detox protocol prior to, and after, the removal of the amalgams that includes taking chlorella (more on chlorella in Tip 2).

SIDE NOTE: **Tips on Improving Oral Health & Preventing Cavities:**

Oil Pulling – an ancient Ayurvedic dental technique to clean, detoxify, remove harmful bacterial and improve gum health. Take 1-2 teaspoons of coconut oil and swish in your mouth for 20 minutes. Then spit the oil in the garbage or toilet, not your sink as the oil can thicken and clog pipes. Finally, rinse your mouth out several times with warm water to rid the oil and toxins that come with it.

Baking Soda – Dip your toothbrush with toothpaste on it into baking soda. Brush your teeth as you normally would. The baking soda helps to remove plaque, prevent tooth decay and whitens your teeth. It also helps to create an alkaline oral pH, which reduces the risk of tooth decay as harmful bacterial require an acidic pH to grow.

Tip 2: Take Chlorella: A freshwater blue-green algae that binds to toxins such as mercury and expels them from your system. You can supplement it in the form of a tablet or powder. You can also buy it in algae form and juice it.

Tip 3: Take Zeolite: A naturally occurring mineral formed from the fusion of lava and ocean water with a unique, negatively charged, crystalline structure, zeolite has a chelation-like effect in removing heavy metals (particularly lead, mercury, cadmium and arsenic), pesticides, herbicides, PCBs, and other toxins from the body. It's taken as a supplement and comes in liquid, powder and capsules.

Tip 4: Patch up with Glutathione: Existing within the body, the amino acid glutathione (GSH) is the most powerful antioxidant free radical scavenger to help eliminate heavy metals. But it's also wise to supplement as most of us today have an overload of heavy metals in our bodies and our glutathione systems are overworked and need support. Glutathione comes in supplement form but the best absorption is with the glutathione patch.

Hydrate
If you increase urine flow, you increase detoxification. To stay hydrated throughout the day, drink:
- Herbal teas made with filtered water
- Juices like celery, cucumbers, and watermelon in season (juice with rind)
- Filtered water to equal half your body weight (128 pounds equals 8 glasses of water, or 64 ounces)

Eat
- Eat raw veggies as they have a high water content, especially celery and cucumbers

- Eat juicy fruits like grapes and watermelon, both great hydrators

Skin - Sweat It, Slough It

The first way to detoxify the skin is to sweat out toxins. You can do this in several ways:

- Exercise
- Infrared sauna or steam
- Hot bath
- Foot bath

The next way to detoxify the skin is by exfoliating. This is done with a vegetable fiber brush, using circular and long strokes towards your navel. Brush for three to five minutes before taking your daily shower. This will slough off dead skin cells, stimulate acupressure points, activate lymphatic drainage, and keep your skin soft and healthy.

Breathe It Out

Detox your lungs with deep breathing. If the breath isn't deep and doesn't reach completely into the diaphragm, the toxins in the bloodstream aren't being transferred over to the outgoing breath.

Boost Lymphatic Drainage

Get the lymph system moving. The lymph system consists of a network of vessels and ducts that move fluid throughout the body, and bring nutrients to the cells and takes waste away from cells. As it lacks its own pumping mechanism, we need to encourage lymphatic drainage. Here's how.

- Exercise
- Get a lymphatic massage

- Take a clay bath
- Use the Chi machine

Get the Right Amount of Sun

We've been made to believe that being out in the sun is bad for you. In truth, you must get your D vitamins from the sun for good health. And the sun's rays are the biggest killer of toxins and the most powerful immune system builder. Even Hippocrates, ancient Greek physician from 400's B.C., was a big advocate of the sun because of its healing properties.

Heliotherapy

Heliotherapy therapy, the use of sunlight as medicine was in its heyday in the 1920's and 1930's. Realizing the power of sunlight to boost the immune system, physicians would wheel patients out onto the hospital sun deck to bake in healing sunlight. Some of the conditions treated included bacterial infections, sepsis, tuberculosis, mood disorders, seasonal affective disorder, skin disorders (acne, psoriasis, etc.). It helped with sleep disorders as well.

Heliotherapy and hospital sun decks disappeared with the discovery of penicillin which marked a new era in medicine and the subsequent widespread use of drug and pharmaceuticals for healing.

Get Enough Sunlight

Sunlight is not dangerous, getting burned is and it ages the skin. The key is to use caution and common sense to avoid getting burned.

To get sufficient vitamin D3, expose your skin for around 20 to 30 minutes daily, preferably before 10 a.m.

and after 4 p.m. Those who are very fair, had excessive past sun exposure or have a history of skin cancer should cover their skin with clothing and wear a wide-brimmed hat during peak hours. Sun and UV (ultraviolet) protective clothing, swimwear and other outdoor products are easily available in stores and online.

SUMMING UP

To stay healthy, you must cleanse internally.
It requires:

- Cleansing the colon and liver
- Removing remove heavy metals from the body by getting the silver out of your mouth and taking supplements like chlorella and zeolite and glutathione
- Staying hydrated
- Sweat and slough off the skin
- Deep breathing
- Boosting lymphatic drainage
- Getting out in the sun

STEP 8
Detoxing from Outside

In this chapter, you'll learn:

- Why you should pay attention to anything that touches your skin.
- Why it's important to replace chemical products with natural, preferably organic products
- Why it's important to open a window whenever possible.
- Tips to improve your indoor quality of life.

Beware of What Touches Your Skin

Synthetic fabrics, bedding and personal care, all contain chemicals that your body will absorb when in contact. Replace them with safe, healthy natural ones.

Clothing

Wear natural fibers, like linen, cotton, wool, silk, bamboo and hemp, as these fabrics allow your skin to breathe. When possible wear organic clothing to avoid exposure to pesticides and chemical dyes.

Avoid clothing that needs to be dry cleaned which is done using toxic chemicals like perchloroethylene -- "perc." Instead look for "organic," "all natural" or "green" dry cleaners that use the following methods: CO_2 cleaning, silicone cleaning, wet cleaning or K4 system.

BEWARE: Polyester clothing and bedding are coated with formaldehyde to resist wrinkling, and emit positive (bad) ions.

Bedding

Sleep on organic cotton or linen sheets or you will be inhaling toxic fumes while you sleep.

Buy an organic cotton mattress or futon as it will breathe and help repel dust mites. It will also keep your body at a more constant temperature.

HELPFUL HINT: A cheap and effective way to clean a mattress is using baking soda. Spread baking soda throughout the entire mattress and rub it in. Let it sit for an hour and then vacuum the mattress. Cleaning with baking soda will help remove odors, dust mites, dirt and contribute to a better night's sleep. Adding several drops of tea tree oil or essential oil such as eucalyptus or lavender to the baking soda before spreading it on the mattress will further enhance detoxification.

You can also place your mattress somewhere inside that will allow direct sunlight, which will further deodorize and kill bacteria naturally.

Personal Care Products

In using skin cleansers and beauty products, the rule of thumb is: if the ingredients of the product were not at some point or at some phase 100% natural or vegetable-sourced, don't put it on your skin. What goes onto your skin goes into your body. Replace synthetic hygiene products with natural, preferably organic ones. These products may include suntan lotions, underarm deodorant, perfumes, colognes, make up, lipstick, cotton pads, tissues, and moisturizers.

Home Clean-Up

Replace commercial cleansers with non-toxic, non-polluting, sustainable, fragrance free and renewable "green," environmentally-friendly household cleaners. A wide array of these products is available at health food stores and some supermarkets. You can also use time-tested natural cleaning products, like vinegar, baking soda, salt, borax, lemon juice, and reusable steel wool. For each of these natural ingredients, *Youtube.com* has a ton of videos showing you exactly how to use them. It seems like everyone is willing to show their natural cleaning secrets.

Home Decoration

From the paint on your the walls to your floor and furniture, most commercial products are laden with dangerous chemicals, including formaldehyde that we all ingest. Some people, who spend numerous hours in new and remodeled homes and offices with much chemical exposure and poor indoor air quality suffer Sick Building Syndrome (SBS). Some of the symptoms reported include headaches, nausea, dizziness, aches, pain, fatigue, irritation to the eyes and throat, runny nose, poor circulation and the list goes on.

To avoid unnecessary exposure, opt to paint your walls with "eco" or "natural" no VOC paint, use natural flooring like wood, bamboo and stone and natural fabrics on your furniture like linen, cotton and bamboo.

The Air You Breathe

Most of us spend the majority of our day indoors, typically with windows closed. This is not good for our health. Air pollutants are two to five times more concentrated inside than in outdoor air, estimates the Environmental Protection Agency.

Stay away from air fresheners including scented candles and toilet deodorizers as they can release chemicals in the air you breathe and have negative health consequences. Unless it's freezing out, try to keep a window open. When possible, use fans, especially ceiling fans and open windows in place of air conditioning. And do let the sun shine in as it is nature's detoxifier.

Here are some tips to clean and improve the indoor air quality you breathe:

Tip 1: Change the filters on your air conditioning and heating units regularly (every 4-6 weeks). Have your home's air duct system professionally cleaned as the air duct system can be a major cause of poor indoor air quality. The National Air Duct Cleaners Association recommends getting your air ducts cleaned every three to five years.

Tip 2: Use a dehumidifier at 30% to 50% to decrease the moisture and prevent mold, mildew and dust mites.

Tip 3: Use a HEPA (high-efficiency particulate air) filter even if you don't suffer from allergens or other pollutants. It cleans the air you breathe.

Tip 4: Test for Radon. Radon is a radioactive, colorless, odorless, tasteless gas that moves through the ground to the air above. More on radon at the Environmental Protection Agency website: www.epa.gov/radon

Tip 5: Buy a Carbon monoxide (CO) detector. CO is a colorless, odorless, and tasteless gas. It's the result of burning fuel in stoves, grills, fireplaces, gas ranges, or furnaces. CO can build up indoors and can be deadly if not detected. Most homes have CO detectors in addition to their fire detectors.

Tip 6: Reduce Electromagnetic Fields (EMF's) and Radio Frequencies (RF's). EMF's and RF's are a result of energy from electrical devices and communications and we are bombarded by them, from power lines and electric appliances to microwaves, vacuum cleaners, hair dryers, compact fluorescent light bulbs, cell phones, wireless computer networks, local wireless networks, wireless radio and television transmissions, cell towers and antennas. While the mainstream view is that exposure is too minimal to be dangerous to our health, daily exposure year after year adds up. The International Agency for Research on Cancer (IARC), (part of the World Health Organization) classified EMF's/RF's as possibly increasing risk of cancer in humans. Wireless phones were associated with the formation of glioma, a malignant brain cancer. Other resources suggest childhood leukemia, Alzheimer's, decreased fertility and decreased melatonin, a powerful human hormone that, if affected, can lead to various cancers, cardio vascular disease, depression and other mood disorders.

While it's difficult to avoid EMF's and RF's, you can take precautions:

Cell Phone Use: Keep cell phones away from your body and head, at least six inches is suggested. Using the speaker phone may not be practical, but is an option. There are companies that specialize in shielded wire earpiece or headsets. Some companies also have devices that can be placed on the phone and claim they reduce EMF's and RF's. Men should not carry cell phones in their pockets as this can reduce fertility. Kids should not use cell phones and pregnant women can wear specific protective clothing to reduce signals while fetus is developing. Low signal areas are actually a health benefit.

While Sleeping: Keep cell phones, computers and other electronic devices away from you when sleeping, including alarm clocks. A battery-operated alarm is better. If you're sleeping on a mattress with coil springs, consider replacing it with an air mattress or memory foam mattress as the coils may act as an antenna that amplifies the intensity of EMF signals. Since you spend roughly a third or your life on a mattress sleeping, it may be a good investment.

Wireless: Replace Wi-Fi routers with ethernet cables and replace other wireless devices with wired devices to reduce signals. During sleep hours or non-use times, turn off router and Wi-Fi.

Laptop: Keep laptop computers off your lap to reduce the negative effects of electromagnetic fields. If you notice a small cylindrical nodule or lump on the end of your computer or monitor cords, these are specifically designed to reduce or filter signal interference. They're called ferrite beads. They can be purchased separately and placed on electronic devices, headsets and earphones to further reduce signals.

Living Area: If you live near power lines, cell phone towers, or a high density of electrical wiring you may want to consider a new location.

Use EMF Reducing Products: A wide variety of products are available designed to reduce EMF and RF signals. They include all types of clothing, wall paints, drywall, room filters, clear window film, protective shields and drapes. To find specific information type in an internet search engine, "Protection from EMF and RF?" This is a topic that is not mainstream, and product resources should be researched.

Tip 7: Green up your home and office. Plants absorb carbon dioxide (the air we breathe out) and release oxygen (the air we breathe in). Using them inside can help detoxify the air. NASA Clean Air Study researched several indoor plants to identify the purification effects of the air in its space facilities and the type of chemical the plant was able to remove. The indoor chemicals removed were formaldehyde, ammonia, benzene, trichlorethylene and xylene. A partial list of the plants included: the Peace lily, Florist's chrysanthemum, English Ivy and Variegated Snake Plant. For the entire list of the plants studied, type NASA Clean Air Study in an internet search engine.

SUMMING UP

- Use natural, preferably organic products for self-care, cleaning and home decoration. If you are using household products that are not natural or organic, you can look up the health and safety information (including the ingredient and the potential health effects). Visit the National Institute on Health's website: https://hpd.nlm.nih.gov
- Bottom line, keep your air clean

STEP 9
Exercise

"Movement is a medicine for creating change in a person's physical, emotional, and mental states."

~ Carol Welch

In this chapter, you'll understand:

- Why the sedentary life is bad.
- How exercise not only helps us stay physically fit but mentally fit as well.
- Why exercise is a natural anti-depressant.
- What different exercises have to offer.

Do you spend your day glued to a chair and staring at a computer screen for hours? Good chance you do. And at night, good chance you're lying flat on your derrier watching TV. But this sedentary lifestyle is unhealthy and unnatural.

Every cell and system in our body is designed for motion. Moving keeps our bodies in shape, our minds sharp and our mood upbeat, as movement feeds our brain and balances out our neurotransmitters.

In truth, there's no end to the benefits of exercise.

Boosts Energy. According to research, the more you exercise, the more energy you have.

Enhances Brain Function. Exercise releases endorphins. These natural high chemicals clear your mind so you can think better, be smarter and remember more.

Enhances Mood. Endorphins also make you feel relaxed and upbeat. In fact, much research has found exercise better at alleviating depression than anti-depressants.

Prevents Disease. Exercise oxygenates the blood, strengthening your heart and helping to prevent a wide spectrum of diseases and illnesses.

Manages Weight. Exercise boosts metabolism, firms the body and helps you shed fat.

Better Joint Health. With increased muscular strength comes better structural support which decreases joint stress.

Deepens Sleep. The excess energy you burn off while exercising makes it a perfect remedy for restless or sleepless nights.

Move. Your life depends on it.

Where to Start

It's always interesting to see the gyms packed full with people at the beginning of a new year or in the spring as summer approaches. Then after a couple months, the gym dies down and goes back to its normal flow.

Why is that?

As someone who's been going to the gym for years, here's my insight: physical pain from overzealousness and mental fatigue.

Imagine starting your New Year's resolution to get back in the gym. You immediately go 100% on every single exercise. You even add more exercises to ensure you've worked out hard enough. The next day you're beyond sore, but it's time to work out again. *Oh no*, you think. And make every excuse why you can't go.

It's not just the physical pain. It's also mental exhaustion from asking so much of yourself.

What's the solution? Make working out easy by making your workout smarter, not harder. Here's how:

Take One Step at a Time

To succeed in making working out a lifestyle, it's critical to get both your mind and your body into the workout together. So instead of going all out, hold back. On your first day back in the gym go so light that you feel you're hardly pushing yourself. Add minimal intensity on each subsequent workout until you reach a comfortable, non-painful level and your workouts become a natural routine. This takes a lot of discipline, but the end goal is results over time.

Also, by not feeling pain you will look forward to going to the gym on subsequent workouts as your mind isn't perceiving the gym as difficult. You'll know when working out is a lifestyle when you start to feel guilty about missing a workout.

And always remember, the competition isn't with your fellow gym mates, but rather with yourself.

Diets and Exercises Don't Work Together

Along with your New Year's resolution to hit the gym, there's a good chance you also started dieting to lose weight. And while this is commendable as long as the diet consists of whole, healthy food, restricting calories actually works against your work outs.

Your body needs enough energy to feed your system to maximize your workouts and exercise programs. If you restrict calories while exercising, your body won't get enough fuel (food) and goes into starvation/survival mode. Your body literally breaks itself down (catabolism) and your own physiology will work against you.

This happens because the muscles are the first source it draws from, not fat. Your body will try to store fat because of the higher calories it can draw from. As a result, you lose muscle and store more fat. To further prevent starvation, you will naturally crave high calorie foods such as fats, sugars, etc. Therefore, it's almost impossible to stick to the diet. Most people end up putting the weight back on in the end.

In place of dieting, institute a good eating plan as highlighted in Steps 3 & 4.

Four Major Types of Exercises:
1. Weight lifting (including weight resistant training)
2. Aerobics (such as running, spinning, elliptical, Stairmaster or swimming)
3. Stretching (including Yoga, Pilates)
4. Plyometrics (including Parkour)

An ideal workout would include all the above, but with an emphasis on lifting weights or weight resistance training.

1. WEIGHT LIFTING/TRAINING

Have you ever observed people in the weight room versus those who just focus on aerobics? You'll see marked difference in the body shape and tone of the two groups. Regardless of sex or age, the weight lifting group is generally in better shape with more lean muscle. One exception is those who apply *high intensity interval training* to their workouts (more on this later).

A BASIC MYTH ABOUT BIG MUSCLES AND WOMEN: Many of my female patients are reluctant to lift weights because they worry about getting big huge muscles. This is a misconception. Unless your family has a history of building large muscles quickly, this really isn't possible. The women in the magazines and on TV with huge muscles have worked immensely on their bodies with stringent weight lifting strategies, including muscle mass building diets and supplementation, and often by taking anabolic steroids or growth hormones.

Benefits to lifting weights:

- Increased overall metabolism
- Increased growth hormone and testosterone, which assists in breaking down of fats and development of muscles
- Improved bone density
- Improved insulin sensitivity and glucose tolerance, which prevents Type II Diabetes
- Creates a longer after burn than aerobic exercises

Improved Metabolism

One of the best ways to speed up your metabolism is lifting weights. The larger amount of lean muscle on your body, the faster your metabolism.

The need to increase metabolism becomes an issue especially as we age. A 2008 study showed that between 20 and 70 years of age, the human body losses 30% of its muscle mass. That's seven pounds of muscle loss every ten years between 20 and 70. The best way to combat this is to lift weights.

How can I get going on a weight lifting routine?

To start, you need to understand the following:

Repetitions: known as reps, these are how many times you lift progressively within a set.

Sets: the number of repetitions you perform for that exercise.

Lifting Exercises by Muscle Groups

The next few pages are diagrams of weight lifting exercises for each muscle group. The muscle will be listed along with the exercises.

The diagrams are just examples of common weight lifting exercises. There are many variations and other exercises to achieve the same result. Depending on the muscle group and exercise goal, you'll usually perform 1-3 exercises in each muscle group. I'll put it all together later in the chapter.

Diagrams of
Muscle Groups and Exercises

LEGS

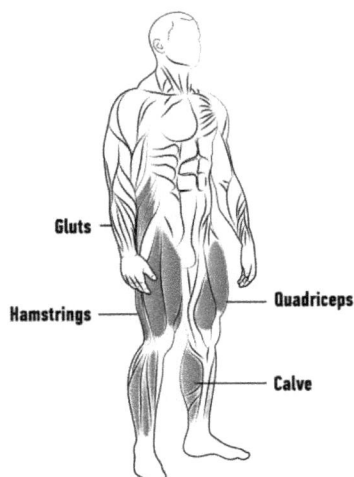

Gluts

Hamstrings

Quadriceps

Calve

SQUATS

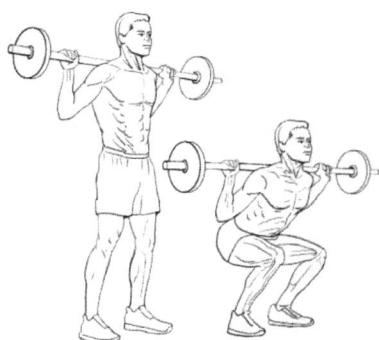

LEG PRESS

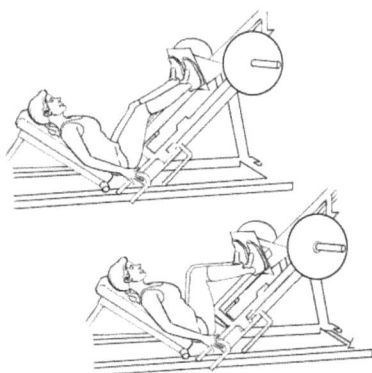

LEG LUNGES

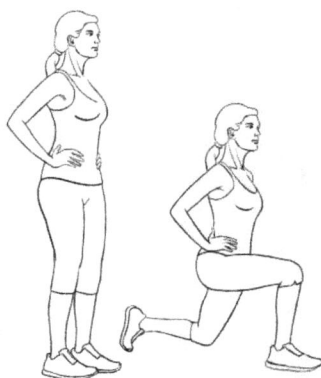

LEGS

SQUATS-NO WEIGHTS

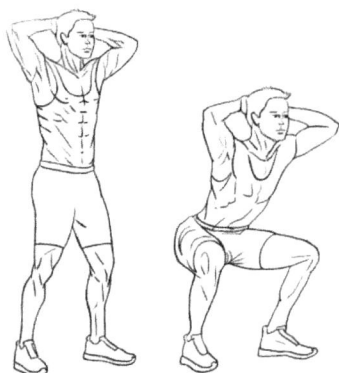

LEG CURLS

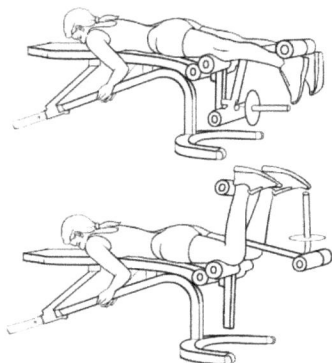

LEG EXTENSIONS

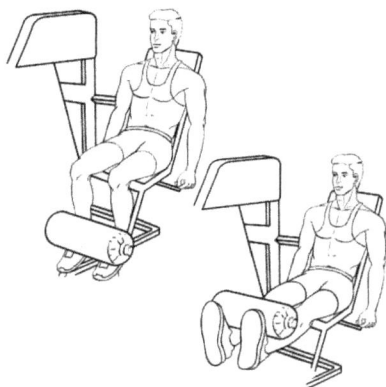

CALF RAISES

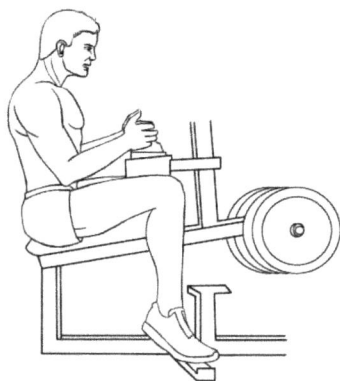

CHEST

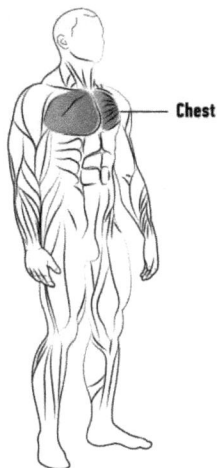

Chest

BENCH PRESS

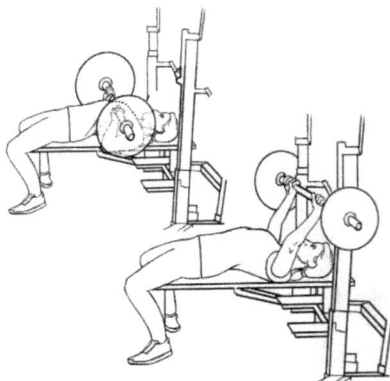

DUMBBELL FLYES

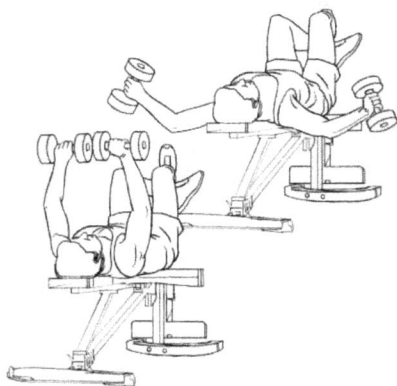

SEATED MACHINE CHEST PRESS

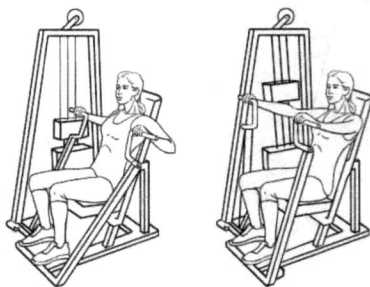

CHEST

MACHINE PEC DECK	PUSH UPS

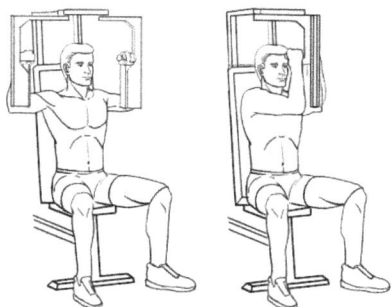

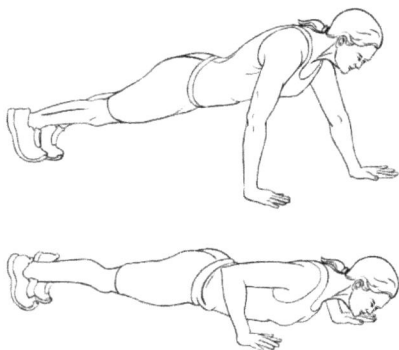

INCLINE PRESS	DECLINE PRESS

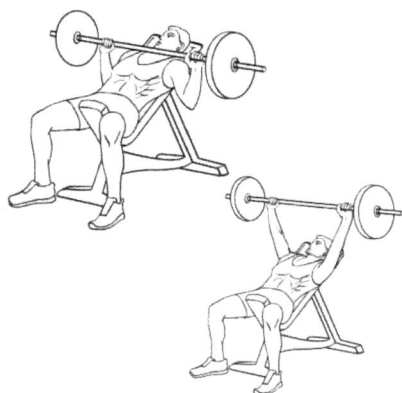

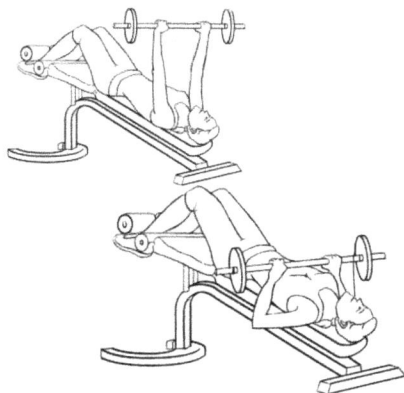

SHOULDERS

Shoulders

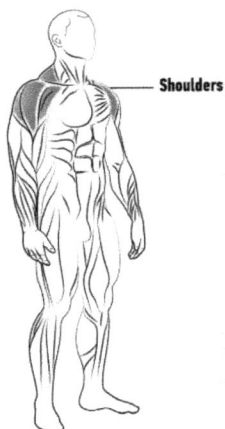

MILITARY PRESS

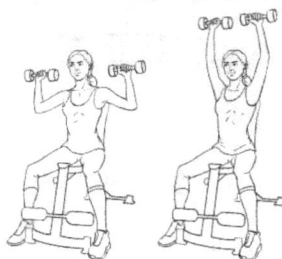

UPRIGHT ROWS

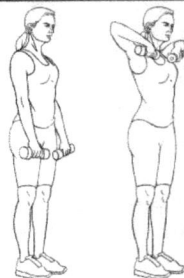

ANTERIOR RAISES

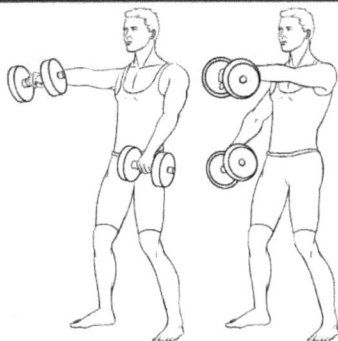

LATERAL RAISES

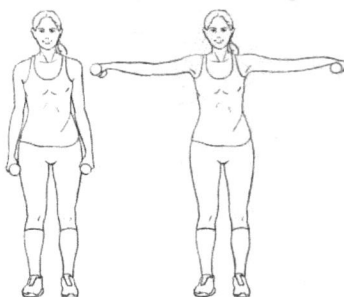

BACK

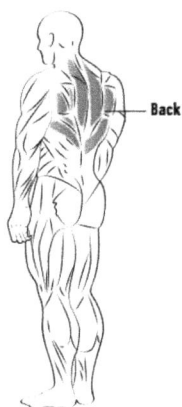

Back

PULL UPS

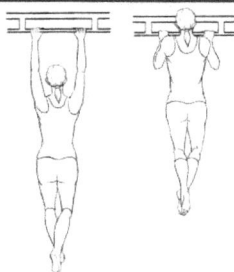

MACHINE LAT PULLS

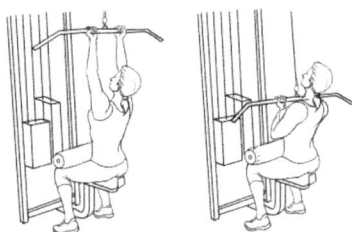

SEATED ROWS

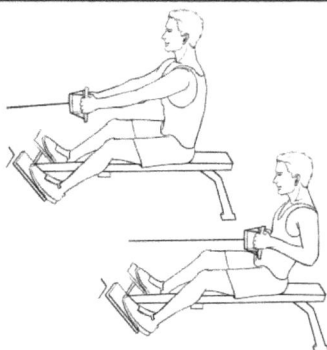

ONE ARM DUMBBELL ROWS

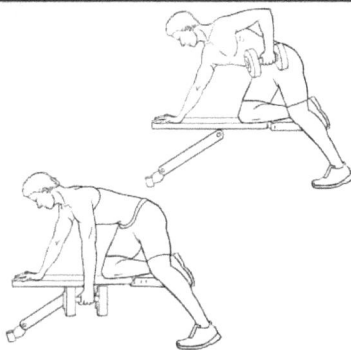

TRICEPS

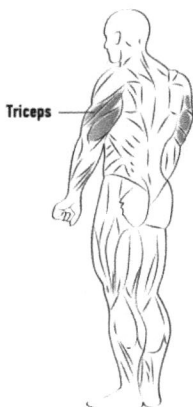

Triceps

TRICEPS PUSH DOWN

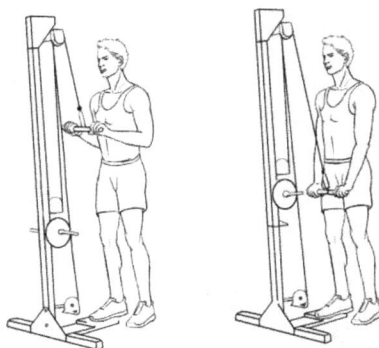

REVERSE CABLE TRICEP PUSHDOWN

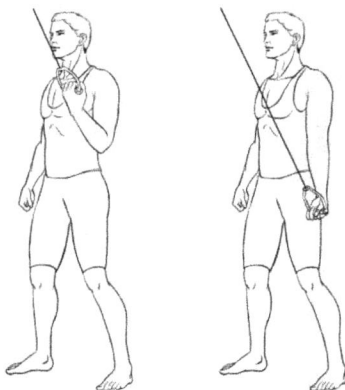

DIPS

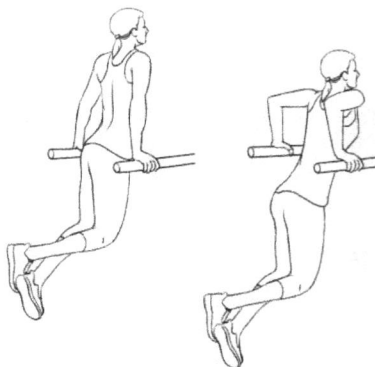

BICEPS

Biceps

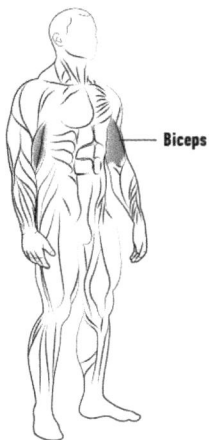

STANDING CURLS

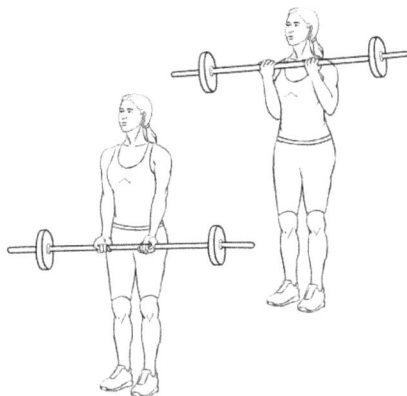

PREACHER CURLS

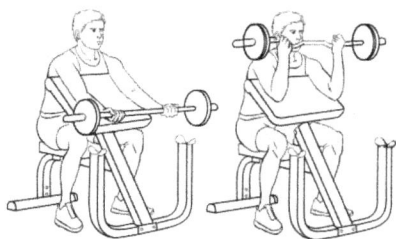

ARM DUMBBELL CURLS

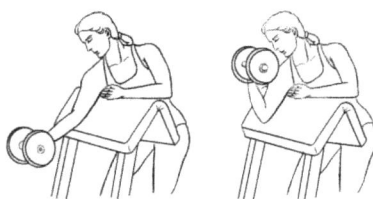

ABS

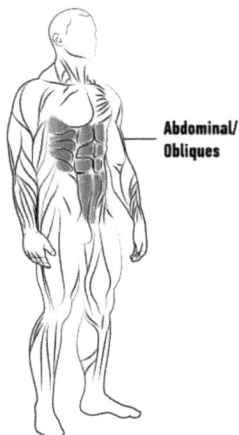

Abdominal/
Obliques

OBLIQUE CRUNCHES

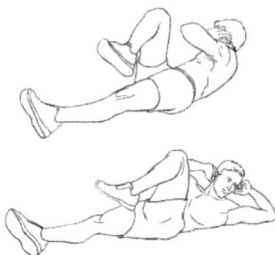

CRUNCHES

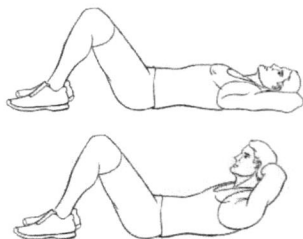

LEG LIFTS

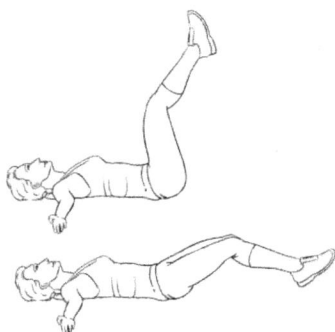

PLANKS

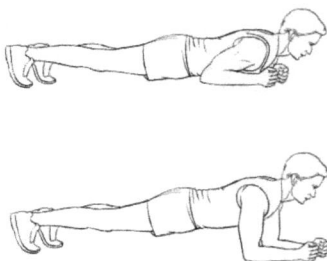

Workout Goals:

Strength & Size - If your goal is to lift weights for strength and size, do lower reps and lower sets (3-4 sets of 6-8 reps).

Tone & Stamina - If you're looking to build tone and stamina, do higher reps and higher sets (4-5 sets of 8-12 reps).

If you want to do a hybrid of the two, be creative and mix it up. This is fun, combats boredom and always tests the muscle.

Length of Time

Depending on your fitness goals, your workout can range from 15 minutes to an hour or more.

Order

The muscles should be worked out according to largest group to the smallest for each day's work out.

The largest muscle group to the smallest are:

- Legs
- Chest
- Shoulders
- Back
- Triceps
- Biceps

Keep in mind the largest muscle groups also indirectly work smaller muscle groups. For example, working out the chest muscles also indirectly works the shoulders and triceps. Another example is if you work out the back, you also indirectly work out the biceps. You get better gains with less effort by organizing similar muscle groups together on the same day. This is a smarter way to workout, not a harder way.

Vary Intensity from Light, Medium, Heavy

If you do more than one exercise for a particular muscle group, make one heavy and the others light or medium. Many new weight lifters make a mistake of lifting heavy for every exercise. This adds to burnout and a lack of gains.

Mix it up

Change up the exercises within the muscle group. For example, if you're working the chest always switch up and change the type of exercises for the chest. Doing so will reduce overuse injuries, build and stimulate new muscles, keep you out of ruts and keep you from plateauing. Changing up the exercises also helps keep you from getting bored as you're always doing something different and in varying parts of the weight room.

Putting it Together

There are a lot of ways to organize your weight lifting routine. Here are some suggestions:

Exercise Example 1

Simple home routine. This is for those with limited time or no access to a gym:

- Squats
- Walking lunges
- Push ups

- Pull ups
- Triceps dips
- Crunches
- Planks

Perform 2-4 days a week.

Perform 3-4 sets for each exercise.

Perform reps to your comfort level and add on as you gain strength and get into a routine.

Mix up the order of exercise and have light, medium and heavy days. For example, squats may be heavy on Monday, light on Wednesday and medium on Friday, whereas push-ups may be light on Monday and medium on Wednesdays and Fridays.

For strength and size try 3-4 sets of 6-8 reps for each exercise; **For tone and stamina** try 4-5 sets of 8-12 reps.

Abdominal exercises can be done 3-5 times per week. Most of your ab development will come from the foods you eat and the intensity of your weight workout.

Exercise Example 2

More complex gym workouts. For those who have access to a weight room and more time to commit to body fitness.

From one workout to the next, switch up the exercises for each muscle and vary the intensity between heavy, medium and light. The exercises listed below are just an example. There are many more exercises to choose from. Keep the order of muscle groups the same, as this is intended to work the larger muscle groups first.

Mon and Thurs

Chest

- Bench press
- Incline press
- Flyes

Shoulder

- Seated military press
- Lateral raises

Triceps

- Push downs
- Dips

Tues and Fri

Back

- Pull ups
- Rows

Biceps

- Curls
- Preacher curls

Wed and Sat

Perhaps one of the leg days is replaced by walking, running, hiking or climbing.

Legs

- Leg press
- Leg extension
- Leg curls

Exercise Example 3

Overall workout for all body parts with people who have limited time, but have access to a weight room.

- Squats, leg curls, leg extensions
- Bench press and/or flyes
- Military shoulder press and/or upright rows
- Dips and/or push downs
- One arm dumbbell curls and/or preacher curls
- Abdominal work

This workout can be performed 2-3 times per week.
Again mix up the exercises for each body part, stay with the order of largest muscle group to smallest and make light, medium and heavy days for each particular exercise.

2. AEROBIC AND CARDIO WORKOUTS

Even though we've spent considerable time laying out the importance of weight lifting, aerobics should not be ignored as there are many benefits:

- Lowered heart rate

  FYI: If resting pulse rate is lowered to 55 beats per minute versus 80 beats per minute that equals 30,000 more beats per minute per day.

- Increased good HDL cholesterol
- Decreased blood pressure
- Increased circulation to the brain
- Aide in detoxification

Nevertheless, if you're doing excessive cardio such as long distance running or spending a lot of time on the stationary bike, there are negatives. Cardiovascular exercises will increase stress hormones such as cortisol and endorphins. Cortisol stimulates appetite and can lead to increased fat storage and slow exercise recovery. It can also decrease testosterone and growth hormone along with suppressing the immune system.

Keep in mind that cardio is important, but balance it with weight lifting and stretching.

High Intensity Interval Training, Burst or Surge Training

A recent workout crave that is in high demand is high intensity interval, burst or surge training.

This training method provides bouts of repeated high intensity exercising, repeated several times over 10-30 minutes followed by less intense recovery time. For example, instead of running for 30 minutes, you apply high intensity burst or surge training for 15 minutes (alternating bursts of sprints with jogging). By doing this, you achieve better results in less time. It might take more discipline, but the net results are more productive workouts.

Benefits of High Intensity Interval Training

- Used for all fitness levels
- Increases aerobic and anaerobic fitness
- Causes muscle building and decrease muscle wasting
- Increases growth hormone and testosterone
- Afterburn effect - burns calories several hours after workout

3. STRETCHING, YOGA, PILATES
Stretching

Mobility and movement are essential to every cell, tissue, organ, and overall body. But as we age, we lose our flexibility. Our range of motion decreases and stiffness increases. By remaining flexible we reduce the chances of injury and joint stress. As the saying goes, "use it or lose it."

The best way to stretch is to hold the stretch for 10 to 20 seconds, rest for 10 seconds and then repeat for 3-4 reps. Never bounce into a stretch as this can lead to unexpected strain/sprains. Always ease into the stretch and hold.

What stretching exercises should you do? That depends on your particular sport or activity. The best way to find stretches for your particular sport or activity is to type it in along with stretches in your favorite internet search engine. For example, "golf stretches" or "gardening stretches."

Yoga

Yoga has become a popular craze in all age groups. And for good reason. There are many benefits. Yoga increases flexibility, muscle tone and strength, improves posture, athletic performance and balance, stretches and stimulates internal organs, and boosts energy. It helps as well with back and neck problems, alleviates stress and gives a sense of wellbeing and peace.

Commit to getting out your mat at home or joining a yoga class.

Pilates

Pilates refreshes mind and body. It helps elongates lean muscles, improves joint mobility and muscle flexibility and reduces back and neck problems. Pilates also works on controlled body movement contributing to improved posture, tone and core strength.

Along with yoga, Pilates also improves proprioception. Proprioception gives us body awareness. In constant feedback to all body parts, proprioception tells us where our feet and hands are in space even without looking. For instance, you can touch your nose and button your shirt without looking.

As we age, we lose proprioception. This is why the elderly will feel unsure of their footing. Both Pilates and yoga slow this loss.

4. PLYOMETRICS

Plyometrics are exercises that involve jumping or jumping like motion, from jumping rope, lunges, burpees, hopping, skipping, jump squats to clapping between push-ups.

Most personal trainers incorporate plyometrics into the beginner's programs all the way to the professional athlete. In fact, most professional sports teams incorporate plyometrics into their workouts because it's an effective way to build explosive power.

***FOR YOUR INSPIRATION:* Parkour** is a training that involves maneuvering through an obstacle course. It involves jumping, rolling, climbing and usually performed around or against buildings, park benches and other structures. You may have seen a social media post of someone who runs into a building then does a flip and then continues to maneuver through varying structures.

Basic Workout Routine

Here's a healthy basic workout routine to cover all the bases:

- Do weight lifting to keep your bones supple and strong
- Bike, dance, swim to keep your lungs working at capacity
- Practice yoga to keep your body young, flexible and strong
- Add a bit of jumping to your daily routine
- Make taking a daily stroll a lifetime habit

How To Keep Your Workouts Consistent

To develop a workout routine that will ultimately become a lifestyle, you must set up a consistent workout routine and especially to motivate you on the days you don't feel like working out. Decide what days you will go to the gym, take a yoga class or bike through the park and keep that schedule.

If you feel tired, not in the mood, don't have the time or something else is calling you, go anyways, even if it means a light workout. If not, not going might become quickly your routine!

Work past your lethargy and get to the gym. You might find, as I have many times, that in spite of poor motivation to work out, you end up actually have an exceptional workout. Make your mantra "I will stick with the routine."

I'm a big advocate of workouts (and sports) for school aged kids. I think it builds character, self-discipline and gives a sense of accomplishment. This gives children lessons in life needed beyond the benefits of workouts.

Tips for Working Out

Tip 1: Consistency in more important than intensity.

Tip 2: Don't grimace while working out; keep your face expressionless to reduce wrinkles.

Tip 3: Be creative. There are several exercises to perform for any given body part. Find those ways to change it up.

Tips 4: Write out your workouts and assign light, medium and heavy exercises within a workout. This combats fatigue and overworked muscles.

Tip 5: Push your muscle load to increase muscle development.

Tip 6: Workout even if you don't feel like it. Make it a light day. Think routine.

Tip 7: Make daily exercise a goal to where you break a sweat.

SUMMING UP

Exercise benefits include:

- Enhancing energy
- Bettering thinking
- Boosting metabolism to manage weight
- Enhancing mood
- Preventing disease
- Deepening sleep

Different exercises serve different purposes including strength, stamina and flexibility.

Step 10
Unwind

"No one can live without experiencing some degree of stress all the time... It is not even necessarily bad for you; it is also the spice of life, for any emotion, any activity causes stress. But, of course, your system must be prepared to take it. The same stress which makes one person sick can be an invigorating experience for another."

~ Hans Selye, M.D.

In this chapter, you'll learn:

- What is the stress response is.
- Why constant stress is bad for health and well being.
- Ways to relax and reduce stress.

Imagine you're camping in the woods when suddenly a bear charges towards your camp site. Your nervous system would react automatically to put you immediately in "fight or flight" mode to ready you to fight the bear, or run. This process unleashes a cascade of effects:

- Adrenals release hormones into your bloodstream targeting muscles and glands and they speed up and contract in preparation of the bear.

- Pupils dilate to better see the bear fast approaching.
- Blood pressure goes up and your heart starts to beat fast.
- Mouth becomes dry and digestive system halts.
- Sex drive, immune system, mental focus all decrease as your body doesn't need these functions right now.

All this happens to fight a true, immediate danger. But in modern life, true danger rarely happens. Rather, we experience constant stress from non-threatening, imagined events like a work deadline, a difficult boss or colleague, a family crisis, a personal conflict.

Fortunately, most of the time, these situations and imagined threats work themselves out and the stress was nothing more than overthinking or over perceiving an event, in essence FEAR (false evidence appearing real).

Nevertheless our body reacts and we get stress related disease like high blood pressure, high cholesterol, digestive problems, sexual dysfunction, depression, and frequent illness, all of which wear down health, and well-being. In fact, some estimate that between 75 - 90% of all physical ailments are the result of mental stress factors. To no surprise, the top selling pharmaceutical medications sold in the U.S. are drugs to counter the symptoms of stress.

Fortunately, many activities can help us alleviate stress.

Breathe Deeply

So many of us are always so rushed that we barely take time to breathe. Little wonder we feel stressed.

Slowing and deepening your breathing is the quickest and most efficient way to change the body from tense to relax. When you take in a deep breath, your body fills with oxygen and the parasympathetic autonomic nervous system takes over to elicit relaxation. You become more aware, settled and balanced.

Here's a quick breathing exercise to deepen and slow breathing.
-Sit or lie in a relaxing position, eyes closed
-Breath in slowly through your nose to a count of four
-Allow your stomach to expand as you breathe in
-Hold your breath for a count of 4
-Release your breath slowly and smoothly, counting to 7
-Repeat 3-5 times

Write It Out

Writing is a cathartic activity to help the mind resolve and work out stressful events and allow the mind to relax from the vicious repetitive thought cycle.

Write down your situation into two columns: pros or positive; cons or negative. Write out all possible pro and con scenarios. Every day add to it.

Avoid Sugar, Caffeine and Alcohol

Sugar can cause mood swings with blood sugar and insulin levels. It may give you a temporary high, but followed by a crash.

Caffeine stimulates the nervous system, which can increase heartbeat and blood pressure, both of which you'd like to eliminate due to stress.

Alcohol also increases heart rate and bloodpressure along with increasing cortisol, a stress hormone. Both caffeine and alcohol are dehydrating and can interfere with sleep. Sleep is critical during stressful times because healing and repair happens while sleeping. Bottom line, choose healthier habits especially when you're under stress.

Other Useful Ways to Handle Stress

- Walk in nature
- Workout and exercise
- Talk it out with friends or family
- Get out of town. Many times, looking at your situation outside your environment contributes to clarity of thought.
- Get a massage or take a hot bath
- Listen to uplifting music, watch inspirational movies and read self-help books
- Go to church or your worship center
- Join an activity group or start one. Groups such as Meetup.com are becoming popular.
- Start a new hobby or learn a new language
- Find things that make you laugh
- Take a break from social media and limit email checking to once per day.
- Change your computer, cell and mobile device screen savers to a tropical beach scene or some other scenery that gives you peace and serenity. Think calm thoughts every time you see it.
- Pick a time to work on relaxation every day

- Learn to say "no" to invites, gatherings and other events that you don't resonate with.
- Eat nutritious meals and stay away from binging on "junk" food

Vitamins that May Help with Stress

- Magnesium
- Vitamin B Complex
- Omega 3
- Melatonin
- Valerian Root
- Turmeric (Curcumin)

SUMMING UP

Stress is inevitable, but how you handle it will be the difference in how your body handles it. Remember to take deep breaths, write it out, avoid perceptions or assumptions of others, let things that you can't control go, avoid sugar, caffeine and alcohol, and follow as many things on the handling stress list as you can.

Step 11
Sleep

"Enough sleep is just as important for good health as nutrition and exercise."
~ Unknown

In this chapter, you'll understand:

- The absolute necessity of quality sleep for physical and mental health.
- How to set up your bedroom to promote sound, restorative sleep.
- What activities interfere with quality sleep.

Life in the hectic world in which most of us live means trying to cram a week into a day. And that means that many of us don't get enough sleep. Yet we must: sleep is absolutely necessary for mental, emotional and physical health. Quality sleep plays a crucial role in immune function, metabolism, memory, learning, and other vital functions.

While asleep, your internal organs work to rejuvenate while your brain files away the day's information. Without a good night's sleep, these processes get compromised and we wake up fatigued and jumpy.

To be most alert and steady the next day, experts generally recommend at least 7-9 quality hours of sleep.

Here are some ways to get better sleep.

Go to sleep & get up consistently at the same time. If you stick to a consistent sleep-wake schedule, you help set your body's internal clock. This will optimize sleep quality.

Go to sleep when tired. If you go to sleep when tired, you will fall asleep more easily and sleep more soundly.

Avoid bright light 2 hours before bedtime. Nighttime light, especially the blue light emitted by electronics from the screen on your phone, tablet, computer, or TV interferes with sleep and body's rhythms by suppressing melatonin, the sleep inducing hormone. Try listening to music or audio books to help you wind down.

Watch the caffeine. A stimulant, caffeine can cause sleep problems up to ten to twelve hours after drinking it. To get a sound sleep, avoid drinking coffee near to sleep time. The same holds true for chocolate which also has caffeine.

Sleep in darkness. The darker your room, the better you'll sleep. You can block light from the windows with heavy curtains or shades, or try covering your eyes with a sleep mask. Move or cover up any electronics that emit light.

Don't eat big meals at night. Heavy, rich foods within two hours of bed will keep you up as fatty foods take much work for your stomach to digest.

Avoid liquids in the evening. Drinking near bedtime can mean frequent bathroom trips throughout the night and especially caffeinated drinks like coffee or soda which act as diuretics.

Create quiet. Try to make your sleeping environment quiet as noise interferes with sleep. If you cannot avoid or eliminate noise from neighbors or people in your household, or from traffic or things like loud air conditioners, try to mask the noise with a fan, a fountain, soothing sounds from an audio source, or white noise. Earplugs may also help.

Keep bedroom cool. Sleeping in a room that is too hot or too cold can interfere with sleep quality. Opt for a slightly cool room with adequate ventilation.

Sleep on a comfortable mattress. Invest in a good, comfortable, long lasting mattress and pillow. To see what best suits you, experiment with different levels of mattress firmness and pillows. I'm an advocate of air mattress systems with a memory foam topper, as this allows you to control the firmness.

Use soothing scents. Dab a few drops of lavender essential oil on the bottom of your feet at bedtime. You'll be surprised how this simple act can calm you into a peaceful sleep.

Let the sun shine in. Try exposing yourself to sunlight as soon as you get up. The light hitting your eyes will help wake you up.

SUMMING UP

Here are some ways to get better sleep:

- Go to sleep & get up consistently at the same time
- Go to sleep when tired
- Avoid bright light 2 hours before bedtime
- Watch the caffeine
- Eat lightly at night
- Minimize liquids in the evening
- Create a quiet environment
- Keep bedroom cool
- Sleep in darkness
- Get a comfortable mattress
- Inhale soothing, natural scents
- Let the sun wake you

PART III
THE RIGHT MINDSET

Step 12
Positive Psychology & Happiness

*"Happiness is the ability to move forward,
knowing the future will be better than the past."*

~ Zig Ziglar

In this step, you'll understand:

- How our thinking affects our thoughts and actions.
- The crucial importance of dispelling false beliefs that leave you stuck in a negative feedback cycle.
- The value of saying affirmations.
- How forgiveness, compassion and gratitude can transform your thoughts and attitude about life.

Dispel False Beliefs

What are you thinking now? Ten minutes ago? Inside your head runs an on-going inner dialogue. These words are extraordinarily powerful and create your reality. They become your self-image and unconsciously guide daily actions and decisions. They create the story of your life.

How do you want that to read? Mostly positive: "I can control my eating." "I can be my ideal weight." "I go for what I want out of life." "I'm capable of doing what I need to do to get ahead." Or mostly negative – "I'm fat, I'll never lost weight, I have no control over my eating."

To take the actions needed to be healthy, vibrant and youthful, your inner dialogue must have a positive message. Now let's look at ways to achieve this.

Challenge Your Beliefs

"Whether you think you can or you think you can't either way you are correct."

~ Henry Ford

Your thoughts come from your beliefs. If they are mostly negative, it's because your beliefs are false and must be changed. Here are some of the most common ones.

"Bad Me"

You demean yourself, call yourself names – "fat, stupid," and focus on what you dislike about yourself.

When someone compliments you, you diminish your positive qualities. For instance, if someone tells you that your stomach looks flatter, you respond with, *"Thank you but my thighs are still fat,"* or *"Yeah, I'm looking good for a fat guy."*

Here's how to change this thinking pattern.

Negative: "No one could love my body."
Change to:
Positive: *"I'm a plus size and that's fine. Many men find natural curves sexy."*

"Poor Me"

Do you feel like a victim of your circumstances – "poor me?" Do you tend to blame something or someone else for your problems? For instance, "If my husband hadn't stuck that chocolate cheesecake in my face, I wouldn't have eaten half the cake."

If so, you let the outside forces control you -- "the devil made me do it." You have what psychologists call an *external locus of control*. You feel that someone or something outside yourself is responsible for how you feel or what happens to you. And so you do little to nothing to change your life because you feel it's out of your hands.

To change, you must feel you are governed by an *internal locus of control* -- that *you* are in charge and in control of what happens to you. Here's how:

Take Charge: Eliminate excuses and denial and take responsibility for your thoughts and actions. *You* spent half your paycheck on a dress you cannot afford. You and no one else! If you blame others, you will continue to make poor choices.

Commit now to the belief that *you* make things happen, not that life is happening *to* you.

You are the master of your fate. What you eat or don't eat, whether you exercise or lie on the couch eating bon bons is in your control. *You must take responsibility!*

HELPFUL TIP: Welcome obstacles as an opportunity for personal growth. To quote Nietzsche, "That which does not kill us makes us stronger." Learn from your mistakes.

Go from Negative to Positive

Negative: "My life is chaos. I have too many errands and responsibilities. How could I possibly find time to exercise?"

Change to:

Positive: "When I can't go to the gym, I'll figure out other ways to get my exercise in like walking upstairs and parking far from the supermarket entrance."

WISE TIP: When you choose an unhealthy food over a healthy one or opt for the couch rather than the treadmill, ask yourself, "Is this serving me?"

Personalization Script

Do you compare yourself to others to determine if you are smarter, better looking, and so forth? Do you believe that what others do or say is a personal reaction to you (egocentricity). For instance, you convince yourself that your sister-in-law didn't come to the family dinner because she dislikes you.

If so, you suffer from personalization or egocentric thinking. Well, guess what? The world has better things to do than to pay attention to your hairstyle, weight, car style and so on. As one of my mentors said to me once, "It's none of my business what other people think of me." You can help get past this adolescent mindset.

1. Change your thought pattern.

Here's how:

Negative: "My son doesn't exercise because I don't. If I were a good mother/father, I would be a better example."

Change to:

Positive: "I'm sure there's lots of reasons why my son doesn't exercise which may have nothing to do with me. Perhaps it's because he feels self-conscious about how much he perspires when he exercises."

2. Step back before reacting. Keep your poise before replying to nasty emails, texts, calls or hand gestures while driving.

Rationalizing Mindset Script

We all make excuses to do that which is bad for us, like over-eat.

Here's how to change this thinking pattern.

Negative: "I had a stressful day at work. I deserve that pizza and bag of potato chips."
Change to:
Positive: "Today was stressful at work but I know how to relax and it's not by eating a pizza and feeling fat and bloated. I will do some deep breathing and meditation instead."

Black or White Script

In this false belief, you judge yourself, your body and your choices as extremely good or bad. If you fall short of your perfectionist ideals, and of course everyone does, you feel like a failure. As a result, you feel that you must do something perfectly or not at all or you're not good enough. Such thinking makes it hard to move forward and greatly impacts lifestyle, making you feel anxious and depressed.

Here's how to change these thinking patterns.

Negative: "If I can't do it perfectly, I won't do it at all."
Change to:
Positive: "My sister is good at everything. But even she's not perfect and I don't have to be either. Good enough is enough."

Practice Daily Affirmations

Affirmations are empowering positive statements that you say to yourself. When you do, you begin to believe that you are healthy, wealthy, young, strong, powerful, loving, happy, and prosperous. Why would this be so? Saying these positive sayings with conviction helps to restructure your brain to believe that anything is possible. Here are some examples of affirmations you might want to say to yourself:

- "I am a winner"
- "I am lovable"
- "I am beautiful"
- "I know how to get what I want in life"
- "I am the master of my fate"
- "I attract fulfilling relationships"
- "I have a healthy and fit body"

Practicing Affirmations

Write your affirmations on a small card in your purse or wallet; put them on post-it notes and/or put them in your mobile device or computer.

Say affirmations out aloud and as if you believe them.

Try to repeat affirmations several times a day. Do this upon awakening or just before going to sleep.

Choose affirmations with the most personal meaning for you.

Avoid Negativity

To help you see the world as half full, rather than half empty, do what you can to avoid negativity in your life.

- Limit time spent watching news
- Seek alternate routes to avoid heavy traffic
- Shop on-line when possible to avoid crowded supermarkets

Seek out Like-Minded People

Try to surround yourself with positive, supportive people who believe in you, encourage you and have similar beliefs and values. Being around people with positive energy will energize, motivate, and inspire you to increase your self-confidence.

Decide to Let It Go

Wayne Dyer, author and spiritual guru told the story of a man sitting next to him on a flight. The man looked miserable. In talking to him, Wayne learned that he was going through a nasty divorce. His wife was going after half of his considerable fortune. Wayne told the man that he could continue following every detail of the divorce and remain miserable. Or he could let it go, let his attorney handle it and take his mind and emotions off it. We all have this choice. Let it go.

Grow Spiritually

Learn to Forgive

When we encounter someone who has wronged us, our bodies tense up and our mind fills with rage. Anger, resentment and desire for revenge engulfs us.

To get past this, we have to change our mindset and make every effort to forgive those who have wronged us. Try to understand that when someone is unkind and heartless, it's from their own unhappiness. Let go of anger and resentment and move on.

Forgive others and forgive yourself for your transgressions; practice self-compassion.

Practice Gratitude

Rather than focus more on what you don't have, focus on all that you do have. Have an attitude of gratitude as the saying goes. Get in the habit of writing daily in a Gratitude Journal. Studies show that simply writing down the things for which you're grateful can make a substantial difference in your overall attitude toward yourself and life.

Every day, find a quiet place to write down three positive things that happened to you that day. These positive things may be as small as someone warmly greeting you to as big as getting married. Continue every day to write three positive things you experienced.

At first you may not see or remember the positive experiences of the day. But after a few days, subconsciously your mind will start to focus on positive experiences and filter out the negative ones effortlessly.

This simple filtering exercise can change your life! You'll start to see the beautiful things that you have been missing.

Practice Compassion

We are all connected. Acts of kindness and compassion will get paid forward, meaning that kind acts will visit you. What we give, we receive. So practice the golden rule always -- what you would not want done to you, you must not do to another. Every day, do at least one kind act. Compliment, volunteer, give up a privilege to help someone out.

SUMMING UP

Choose Your Words Carefully. Inside your head is an on-going inner dialogue that creates the story of your life. When you begin to think positively, you will change the script that runs through your head and your self-image.

Challenge Your Beliefs. False beliefs prevent us from taking responsibility for our lives, limiting our true potential and success. Challenge your false beliefs by reframing them.

Practice Daily Affirmations. Affirmations are powerful positive statements - words that you *consciously* choose to speak to empower yourself.

Practice forgiveness, compassion and gratitude. Daily, write down three things positive things that happened.

STEP 13
Mindfulness Meditation

"There's more to life than increasing its speed."
~ Gandhi

In this chapter, you'll understand:

- The many benefits of mindfulness meditation
- How to practice every day mindfulness
- The importance of doing a sit-down meditation

If you are like most, you speed through the day on autopilot, stuck largely inside your head in on-going mind chatter that, for many is mostly negative. Life sails past you as time flies and never comes back. Is it any wonder that many people turn to food, sex, alcohol, drugs, TV, internet as a diversion to numb discomforting emotions and a means of temporary comfort?

You can change this by becoming mindful. Mindfulness meditation means focusing on the present and living in the moment, putting thoughts aside and savoring pleasures as they occur. This frees you from regrets about the past, which causes depression, and worries about the future which causes anxiety.

Mindfulness Benefits

The benefits of mindfulness meditation are greater than any benefit a pill can ever give you.

Here are some, but by no means all benefits of meditation:

- Reduces stress, anxiety and depression; improves concentration and memory
- Relaxes you by lowering oxygen consumption, decreasing respiratory rate, slowing heart rate, decreasing levels of blood lactate and reducing muscle tension
- Lowers cholesterol levels, reduces risk of cardiovascular disease, and improves flow of air to the lungs resulting in easier breathing and asthma relief

Practicing Mindfulness or Being Present

Every minute of your life, you can practice mindfulness, wherever you are or whatever you are doing. Here are some ways:

Become aware of your body when you are standing in line at the supermarket, filling up your gas tank or washing your face. Notice your breathing, how you are sitting or standing, tension in your muscles. When thoughts enter your mind, observe them neutrally and then let them go.

Take a walk in the park, along the seaside or ocean and focus on just the experience of walking. Experience everything around you as if for the first time.

Focus attention on the grass, trees, birds, water, sand. Notice subtle changes of sounds, ambient scents and the sensation of your feet touching the ground. Become aware of your surroundings. Feel the sun's warmth on your face, feel your hair blowing in the wind. Hear animals in nature, whether it's a squirrel gathering food or a bird chirping.

HELPFUL HINT: Routine in our daily life inhibits our ability to perceive the wonderful things around us mindfully. The solution is breaking out of routine as much as possible and continually seek to experience something new. For example, instead of going to or from work the same way, find different routes and switch it up.

Meditation

Once a day, or more if you wish, set aside at least 10-15 minutes to do a formal meditation. Here's how:

Find a space without distractions. Sit in a comfortable position or lie down. Close your eyes and focus on your breath, your third eye (space between your eyebrows), or a candle flame or repeat a mantra, a sacred word or words of your choice like "om, love, peace." It also helps to listen to and focus on quiet, meditative music.

Become still and notice the rise and fall of your chest, and how your breath comes in and out through your nose. Breathe slowly and deeply. If thoughts enter your mind about the future or the past invade your mind, focus on your breath, the movement of your diaphragm, or some other random noise nearby.

Slowly open your eyes and notice how your breathing is slower and your muscles more relaxed.

A good time to quietly meditate is first thing in the morning to jumpstart your day or before retiring to help wind down and help you relax into a quiet sleep.

If meditation is new to you, purchase a guided mediation audio. Most of them will talk you through meditation with serene music in the background. The list of meditation audio subjects can vary and includes: anxiety, depression, happiness, clarity, peace of mind, deep relaxation, sleep, stress, healing, meditation for beginners and the list goes on. You can buy online or listen for free by typing "guided meditation audio" in your favorite web browser or on YouTube.com.

SUMMING UP

Become mindful. Live in the present. You can do this throughout the day when you don't have to be engaged in thinking, like waiting in line at the supermarket.

Meditate. Practice a daily sit down meditation to learn how to gain control over your thoughts.

STEP 14
Goal Setting, Visualization & Vision Board

*"Imagination's everything. It is the preview
of life's coming attractions."*

~ Albert Einstein

In this chapter, you'll understand:

- Why it's important to set goals.
- How visualizing your goals will help you to better achieve them.
- How a vision board will inspire you.

We all have goals in life that we hope we can achieve. Yet how many of us do achieve them? Not many. Don't be part of this unfortunate statistic. Here are ways to better insure that you will achieve your goals for healthy living:

One Step at a Time

Some people can decide they will do something and go headlong into doing so and stick with it. But this is the rare bird. Most people need to slowly transition into a new lifestyle or the change can feel overwhelming. So don't think you have to dive into it. Instead, think of making a gradual change and taking baby steps. Every journey begins with the first step.

To help you do this, decide you will make one change for each day of the week. Increase this change each week to two days, three days, and so on until you have fully embraced a new healthy lifestyle. For instance:

WEEK ONE:

Monday: Replace diet coke with a healthy drink like coconut water

Tuesday: A 10-minute meditation upon waking

Wednesday: Smoothie for breakfast

Thursday: Gym workout in the evening

Friday: Huge salad for lunch

Saturday: Gluten free day

Sunday: Progressive relaxation before going to bed

WEEK TWO:

Monday: Replace diet coke with healthy drink like coconut water; huge salad for lunch

Tuesday: 10-minute meditation upon waking; gluten free day

Wednesday: Smoothie for breakfast; replace diet coke with healthy drink like coconut water

Thursday: Gym workout in the evening; progressive relaxation before going to bed

Friday: Huge salad for lunch; 10-minute meditation upon waking

Saturday: Smoothie for breakfast; gluten free day

Sunday: Huge salad for lunch; progressive relaxation before going to bed

WEEK THREE:
Increase each activity to three days and repeat this pattern.

By the end of seven weeks, you are locked into your new lifestyle. At this point, add a new activity each week. By the end of six months, you will fully embrace a healthy, holistic lifestyle.

FYI: There is a caveat. As you may know, it takes 21 days to make an action into a habit. If you're not doing it every day it will take longer. Don't worry. By week seven or perhaps sooner, you will be implementing daily changes. Of course, any time you feel that you can handle speeding things up, do so. For instance, if by the third week, you feel you can forego having diet coke forever, go for it!

HELPFUL ADVICE: Of course, some things you can start out doing daily like taking a multivitamin or washing your clothes with natural detergent.

Write Out Your Goals

Years ago, I attended a seminar and heard a speech by Mark Victor Hanson, coauthor of the popular *Chicken Book for the Soul* series and bestselling self-help author. He challenged us to write "101 Lifetime Goals." Game on, I wrote all my 101 goals. Years later, I found this list again. I was in shock with disbelief. I had accomplished many of those goals!

How many of us have had a challenge, wrote it out, slept on it and voilà -- there's our answer and solution.

Writing out both personal and professional/business goals gives you an inner guide and map to set your course.

It's like programming a computer. If you write the software, the computer will perform the task. If you write down your goals (writing the software), your creative right brain and analytic left brain (the computer) will find a way to make your goal a reality.

If you ink it, you'll think it and your conscious and unconscious mind and inner wisdom will find a way to make it happen.

For the upcoming year, write out your goals. List them out. Do the same for your lifetime goals.

For the previous year, write out your biggest successes or things that you accomplished that made your year. Write what you learned (personally and professionally) and how you grew from the previous year. This can be as brief or extensive and detailed as you'd like. You're creating your future.

Visualize Your Goals

The next step in helping you achieve your goals is by visualizing them.

How effective is visualization? Try this. Close your eyes and picture yourself biting into a lemon. What happened? Good chance you started salivating.

Creative visualization is a powerful and rapid means to changing your thinking. Just by seeing in your mind's eye what you want to achieve, whether it will be to become healthier, richer, thinner, nicer, sexier or more loving, visualization will help you know what it would feel like and make it more likely you will take the steps needed to fulfill your dreams.

Visualization's Power

What makes visualization so powerful? The brain cannot distinguish from an activity we visualize from one in which we actually go through the motions. In fact, visualizing something happening holds as much weight as practicing with your body. If you imagine yourself pressing that weight just beyond your comfort level, you will feel your muscles being pushed and fatigued.

Years ago, psychologist Alan Richardson from Australia tested three random groups of basketball players and their ability to make free throws. He performed a baseline performance first, then after 4 weeks checked each group for improvements. The first group practiced shooting free throws for 20 minutes, 5 days a week. The second group only visualized themselves making free throws for that same period of time. The third group neither practiced nor visualized. To their astonishment, the visualization group not only improved, but were almost as good (23%) as those who actually practiced (24%).

So powerful is visualization that top performers in every field, from athletes to CEO's, use it to prepare for a big event. This helps them cultivate the sensation of how it will feel when they win before taking that important step on the field, court or track. Before a fight, Muhammad Ali always pictured himself victorious, while Michael Jordan always saw the last shot in his mind before he threw a hoop. Here's some tips on how to visualize goals:

Imagine Every Step

Picturing every step will help the image come more alive for you.

Get Detailed

See images in exquisite detail. The more vivid, the better the visualization will work for you.

Add Sensations

Visualize not only mental imagery but all five senses. Imagine that you are hearing, smelling, tasting, touching and seeing.

Be Positive

Visualize your images with the cup half full, not half empty. If you wish to lose 20 pounds, picture yourself thin and firm.

Create a Vision Board

The vision board is a visual of what you want in life. Having one helps you attract and manifest the things you want to be, do or have, the idea of which became especially popular after the book and movie *The Secret*.

To make a vision board, cut and paste those images you want to manifest on a document, print it and look at it often. Some prefer to cut those images from magazines onto paper or poster board. In either case, the concept is the same. You want to visualize those things that you want to make reality.

I personally have a folder in my computer called, *Personal Growth*. Under this folder I have my goals, affirmation and my vision board separated by the year. I encourage you to do the same.

SUMMING UP

- Setting goals are very important to help you with a game plan on changing your lifestyle and life.
- Two things that really help in setting goals is to go at it slowly, one step at a time and to visualize what you want for yourself. Remember to ink it and think it.
- Create a vision board to manifest your desires.

Step 15
Putting it Altogether – Your Health Plan

Now that you're (hopefully) all fired up about your health plan, you might wonder how it will actually get played out. Once you've got your new lifestyle changes in place, what will a typical day look like?

Let's take a peek:

Awakening

- Drink water with lemon squeezed in it.
- Do a brief 10-minute meditation to start your day. Finish it by visualizing your goals(s) for the day. Set your intention to make every effort to replace negative thoughts with positive ones.

Morning

- Have a green smoothie for breakfast. Take your supplements.
- While brushing your teeth, practice mindfulness by focusing on the sensation.
- Look in the mirror and say five positive affirmations to yourself.
- Exercise depending on your schedule. If you have the time, start out with a run, a workout at the gym, or a yoga class.

Mid-Morning

- Have a healthy snack like raw nuts or a piece of fruit. Sit outside to eat it so you can get sunlight and your vitamin D.
- Take a moment, close your eyes and do some deep breathing.

Lunch

- Have a huge salad for lunch. Add a rainbow of vegetables. Throw in some fermented veggies.

FOR YOUR HEALTH:

Completely avoid the following:

- Gluten
- Pasteurized dairy
- Artificial sweeteners such as Aspartame
- Flavor enhancers such as MSG (monosodium glutamate)
- Non-Organic food which can contain pesticides, herbicides, hormones, and antibiotics.
- Meat overload
- High-allergen food such as milk, wheat, corn, and soy.

Mid-Afternoon

- Retreat to a quiet place and do a quick 10-minute body scan to help you relax and get through the rest of the hectic day.
- While commuting home, switch it up and find a new route. Observe the new experience.

- Go the gym and do an end of the day workout. While there, show kindness by complimenting someone.
- Do an infrared sauna if your gym has one available.
- Have a healthy snack. No processed food! Drink something fermented like kombucha or kefir.

Dinner

- Eat dinner 3-4 hours before going to bed.
- Eat a dinner that consists of only whole food like brown rice, steamed veggies and beans, or free-range chicken breast with a baked sweet potato and steamed spinach. Be sure and add some fermented food, like kimchi.
- For desert, try some fruit and nuts, like a banana with walnuts and cocao powder mixed in.

Evening

- Take a walk through nature to help you unwind and digest your food.
- Do an infrared sauna if you have a home unit or one at your gym.
- Write out three to five things that happened to you today or for which you feel grateful.

Going to Sleep

- Put lavender essential oil on the bottom of your feet.
- Do progressive relaxation to wind down into sleep.

SUMMING UP

- Eat fruits and vegetables and buy them organic and raw if possible.
- Don't over-cook your meals and stay away from microwave cooking. Drink green vegetable mix or organic dark leafy drinks. Drink filtered water and avoid tap water.
- Do nutritional cleansing and detoxing.
- Avoid drugs, alcohol and smoking.
- Exercise 3 to 6 days per week.
- Enjoy sunshine without overdoing it.
- Protect yourself from EMF and RF pollution
- Create good sleeping habits in a good sleeping environment.
- Handle stress in positive ways and avoid negative emotions.
- Get out in nature or the beach, be present, enjoy breathing the fresh air.
- Take time to let the mind relax and meditate.
- Develop trusting and loving relationships.
- Have gratitude.
- Write goals, affirmations and create a vision board.

"Write it on your heart that every day
is the best day in the year."
~ Ralph Waldo Emerson

NOW IT'S YOUR TURN TO WRITE OUT YOUR HEALTH PLAN:

Vitamin & Supplementation List (list in priority)

1._____

2._____

3._____

4._____

5._____

6._____

7._____

Food and Meal Preparation
List several combinations and rotate from day to day. Remember the priority of carbohydrates, fats and proteins.

Breakfast:
_____
_____

Mid-morning Snack:
_____
_____

Lunch:
_____
_____

Healthy Snack:
_____
_____

Dinner:

_____

_____

Healthy Snack:

_____

_____

Weight Training & Exercise
Weights:

_____

_____

Cardio:

_____

_____

Stretches:

_____

_____

To Do List (Update Daily)
1._____
2._____
3._____
4._____
5._____

List positive affirmations and say them aloud daily.

_____

_____

_____

_____

When experiencing stress over a situation or decision, write out the pros and cons for each circumstance.

Pros_____ Cons_____

_____   _____

Goals

In the upcoming year:

What are my goals?

_____

_____

_____

_____

In the previous year:

What was my biggest successes?

_____

_____

_____

_____

What did I learn?

_____

_____

_____

_____

How did I grow personally and professionally?

_____

_____

_____

_____

List 3 positive things that happen to you today (gratitude list). Update daily.

1._____

2._____

3._____

List 1 or 2 things you did anonymously to help someone or a cause.

1._____

2._____

In Conclusion

"We never know how far reaching something we think, say, or do today will affect millions of lives tomorrow."

~ BJ Palmer

I know a wise older man who grew up in a hardworking family. He had to work exceptionally hard for everything he had.

In his younger years, he had the opportunity to go to college, but only after serving in the military. He served in the United States Army and was stationed in Japan.

After active duty and graduating from college, he worked as a Soil Conservationist for the U.S. government until his retirement. With years came knowledge, experience and wisdom.

He is my father. Here are his 16 principles of life:

1. Don't Lie
2. Don't Steal
3. Develop Self Discipline
4. Develop Determination and Self Esteem
5. Show Respect to Other People
6. Volunteer to Help People as this will Bring Reward
7. Stay away from Smoking
8. Stay away from Alcohol
9. Stay away from Drugs
10. Select Good Friends who really Care for you
11. Happiness Leads to Success

12. Religion is the Foundation of Life
13. Set a Goal as a Destination for Life
14. Try to be better than Most People in One Thing (one doesn't have to be good at everything).
15. Your Family is an Anchor in Life and when things get you down and things get tough - your Family can be counted on to Always Help You.
16. Keep Trying - Never give up. You will Always Rebound.

~ Olin Fimreite

This now ends our journey together. I do hope you feel charged up and positive about starting your new healthy, anti-aging lifestyle.

To a long, healthy, happy life!